Pediatric Sinusitis

Pediatric Sinusitis

Editor

Rodney P. Lusk, M.D.

Director and Otolaryngologist in Chief
Division of Pediatric Otolaryngology
St. Louis Children's Hospital
Washington University
St. Louis, Missouri

Raven Press ✺ New York

Raven Press, Ltd., 1185 Avenue of the Americas, New York, New York 10036

© 1992 by Raven Press, Ltd. All rights reserved. This book is protected by copyright. No part of it may be reproduced, stored in a retrieval system, or transmitted, in any form or by any means, electronic, mechanical, photocopying, recording, or otherwise, without prior written permission of the publisher.

Printed and bound in Hong Kong.

Library of Congress Cataloging-in-Publication Data

Pediatric sinusitis / editor, Rodney P. Lusk.
   p. cm.
   Includes bibliographical references and index.
   ISBN 0-88167-894-5
   1. Sinusitis in children.   I. Lusk, Rodney P.
   [DNLM: 1. Chronic Disease—in infancy & childhood.   2. Sinusitis—
in infancy & childhood.   3. Sinusitis—physiopathology.
   4. Sinusitis—therapy.   WV 340 P371]
   RF425.P44   1992
   618.92′212—dc20
   DNLM/DLC
   for Library of Congress   91-45670
                                                                        CIP

The material contained in this volume was submitted as previously unpublished material, except in the instances in which some of the illustrative material was derived.

Great care has been taken to maintain the accuracy of the information contained in the volume. However, neither Raven Press nor the editor can be held responsible for errors or for any consequences arising from the use of the information contained herein.

Materials appearing in this book prepared by individuals as part of their official duties as U.S. Government employees are not covered by the above-mentioned copyright.

9 8 7 6 5 4 3 2 1

Contents

Contributors

Thomas E. Herman, M.D. *Mallinckrodt Institute of Radiology, Washington University School of Medicine, 510 South Kingshighway Boulevard, St. Louis, Missouri 63110*

Rodney P. Lusk, M.D. *Department of Otolaryngology, St. Louis Children's Hospital, and Washington University School of Medicine, 400 South Kingshighway Boulevard, St. Louis, Missouri 63110*

William H. McAlister, M.D. *Mallinckrodt Institute of Radiology, Washington University School of Medicine, 510 South Kingshighway Boulevard, St. Louis, Missouri 63110*

Harlan R. Muntz, M.D. *Department of Otolaryngology, St. Louis Children's Hospital, 400 South Kingshighway Boulevard, St. Louis, Missouri 63110*

T. S. Park, M.D. *Department of Neurosurgery, St. Louis Children's Hospital, and Washington University School of Medicine, 400 South Kingshighway Boulevard, St. Louis, Missouri 63110*

David S. Parsons, M.D., F.A.A.P., F.A.C.S., Colonel USAF *Department of Otolaryngology, Wilford Hall Medical Center, Lackland Air Force Base, Texas 78236*

Stephen H. Polmar, M.D., Ph.D. *Professor of Pediatrics and Molecular Microbiology, Washington University School of Medicine, and St. Louis Children's Hospital, 400 South Kingshighway Boulevard, St. Louis, Missouri 63110*

Gail G. Shapiro, M.D. *Clinical Professor of Pediatrics, University of Washington School of Medicine, and Northwest Asthma & Allergy Center, 4540 Sandpoint Way NE, Seattle, Washington 98105*

Raymond G. Slavin, M.D. *Department of Internal Medicine and Microbiology, Division of Allergy/Immunology, St. Louis University School of Medicine, 1402 South Grand Street, St. Louis, Missouri 63104-1028*

Lawrence Tychsen, M.D. *Department of Ophthalmology, St. Louis Children's Hospital, and Washington University School of Medicine, 400 South Kingshighway Boulevard, St. Louis, Missouri 63110*

Ellen R. Wald, M.D. *Department of Pediatrics, University of Pittsburgh School of Medicine, Children's Hospital of Pittsburgh, 3705 Fifth Avenue, Pittsburgh, Pennsylvania 15213*

Franz J. Wippold II, M.D. *Mallinckrodt Institute of Radiology, Washington University School of Medicine, 510 South Kingshighway Boulevard, St. Louis, Missouri 63110*

Gerald Wolf, M.D. *University HNO-Clinic, Auenbruggerplatz 20, A-8010 Graz, Austria*

Preface

Children with persistent purulent rhinorrhea, cough, and nasal congestion are no longer considered variants of normal. Chronic sinusitis increasingly is being recognized in many such children by pediatricians, pediatric allergists, family practitioners, and otolaryngologists. Increased awareness has resulted in more interest in the diagnosis and management of children with chronic sinusitis.

Pediatric chronic sinusitis is not completely understood and as a multifactorial disease is particularly difficult to diagnose. The authors of this book—established pediatric sub-specialists and surgeons—summarize the literature and offer the benefit of their experience in their areas of expertise. Thus, this book presents the current knowledge of the pathophysiology and the medical and surgical management of pediatric chronic sinusitis.

Primary-care physicians and pediatricians will find particularly useful the chapters on pathophysiology and associated diseases such as allergy, asthma, and immune deficiencies, as well as the extensive chapter on radiology of the pediatric sinuses. The otolaryngologist will likely profit most from the chapter detailing surgical management. Although all surgical modalities used to treat pediatric chronic sinusitis are reviewed, the focus is on endoscopy. Separate chapters are dedicated to bacteriology and medical management of pediatric chronic sinusitis.

Perhaps the most important purpose of this book is to address the issues involved in the surgical management of pediatric chronic sinusitis. I have become convinced that surgical procedures used in children should be as conservative as possible yet should clear the sites of obstruction. The approach described by Dr. Messerklinger and popularized by Drs. Stammberger and Kennedy make the most sense to me because this technique is designed to remove only the diseased tissue and leave intact, as much as possible, the normal anatomy. As Dr. Stammberger noted in the preface to his book *Functional Endoscopic Sinus Surgery*, "functional endoscopic surgery in children requires expert knowledge and experience and we strongly recommend that novices not start with pediatric cases." I concur with his view and hope this book will help delineate the developing expertise and knowledge in this area.

Rodney P. Lusk

Acknowledgments

Most individual goals are accomplished only with the dedicated assistance of others. The compilation of this book is no exception. It depended on the encouragement, efforts, and sacrifices of both colleagues and family.

First of all, I am indebted to my teachers and instructors throughout my training. In particular, I am grateful to Dr. David Kennedy and Dr. Heinz Stammberger for their outstanding courses, in which I learned the principles of conservative sinus surgery and was given the opportunity to dissect countless adult cadavers. A special thanks also goes to Ellen MacDonald and Hans Steinmann for their assistance in developing the pediatric sinus instruments with Karl Storz. I am grateful for the tolerance of Tammie Hoefft, who endured the early procedures performed without proper instrumentation, and to Dr. Stan Thawley who held my hand during those first few procedures. I am also grateful for the open exchange of ideas with my colleagues and close personal friends, Dr. Harlan Muntz and Dr. David Parsons. I would like to express my appreciation as well to an overworked yet cheerful and stable administrative staff composed of Marilyn Crawshaw, Judy Rickert, and Patty Caruso.

Finally and most important, from the depths of my heart, I thank my wife, Donna, and my children, Tara and Adam, for their love and support. It is to them that I dedicate this book. I pray that I will now be able to give them more of my most precious possession, my time.

Rodney P. Lusk

Pediatric Sinusitis,
edited by R. P. Lusk,
Raven Press, Ltd., New York © 1992.

CHAPTER 1

Signs and Symptoms of Chronic Sinusitis

Harlan R. Muntz and Rodney P. Lusk

Sinusitis varies considerably in its presentation (1–3), and in children the disease and its signs and symptoms are poorly understood. Older children, like adults, will complain of localized symptoms such as pain, tenderness, and pressure. In parts of the country it is not unusual for patients to describe "sinus problems" as allergy-related symptoms. The symptoms of sinusitis overlap with those of allergy, nasal airway obstruction, and other less obvious processes, often making diagnosis difficult. To diagnose any disease, of course, one must review carefully the symptoms related by the patient and add to that the information obtained through physical and laboratory examinations.

Physicians vary in their understanding of sinus disease and their ability to accurately diagnose sinusitis. Table 1.1 is a summary of data collected in a mail survey conducted with pediatricians in the St. Louis area. The purpose of the survey was to determine the prevalence of sinus disease in children as perceived by the primary care providers. Each physician was asked how often he or she saw children with acute sinusitis, recurrent acute sinusitis, and chronic sinusitis. The definitions of acute, chronic, and recurrent sinusitis were left to the interpretation of the pediatrician. The results were surprising because of the wide range of differences in reported occurrences.

The two physicians reporting the highest and lowest numbers of patients with sinusitis are both excellent pediatricians with busy clinical practices and are active on the staff of a university-affiliated children's hospital. They are similar in age and, as far as could be ascertained, have similar patient populations. The variance in the numbers of cases reported for acute sinusitis (1 versus 120 per month) could be accounted for by faulty recollection or an actual difference. Such

a large difference, however, is more likely due to a lack of agreement on what constitutes sinusitis in children. One would expect that neither the highest nor the lowest number is accurate, but something in between is closer to the truth. Thus the incidence and prevalence of acute and chronic sinusitis remain to be defined and will require more specific study.

In the same survey, the respondents were asked how they made the diagnosis of sinusitis. Table 1.2 displays the results. Not surprisingly, the most important information used in the diagnosis was not a laboratory test or radiograph but clinical judgment. This reaffirms the need to understand and define the signs and symptoms of the disease as clearly as possible.

A difficulty in basing the diagnosis on clinical judgment is that the history must be obtained from children who cannot articulate their symptoms or from parents who may exaggerate them. A parent who desperately wants a perfect child may shudder at a runny nose, while parents who have children in day-care settings may expect to see such problems. If there is a strong family history of allergy, symptoms may be described as allergic symptoms, and the infectious nature of the disease may be overlooked. Because many young children are unable to express their own complaints, one must often act as an investigative reporter and seek out the symptoms of sinusitis.

H. R. Muntz and R. P. Lusk: Department of Otolaryngology, St. Louis Children's Hospital, St. Louis, Missouri 63110.

TABLE 1.1. *Presumed incidence of sinus disease seen in pediatric practice[a]*

Disease	Cases reported/month	
	Mean	Range
Acute sinusitis	18	1–200
Recurrent sinusitis	13	4–100
Chronic sinusitis	7.5	1–40

[a] These data came from a survey conducted with 45 pediatricians in the St. Louis, Missouri, area.

TABLE 1.2. *Basis for diagnosing sinusitis*

Basis	Most important	Important	Occasionally important	Total
			Number of responses	
Clinical judgment	20	12	3	35
Sinus series radiographs	16	13	3	32
Waters' view radiographs	8	6	3	17
Nasal smear	—	3	—	3
Anterior rhinoscopy	—	2	2	4
Transillumination	—	2	2	4
CT scan	1	1	3	5

Table 1.3 differentiates the symptoms of acute and chronic sinusitis (4). Table 1.4 presents the symptoms most frequently used to diagnose chronic sinusitis by the pediatricians responding to the survey. Table 1.5 gives the symptoms of chronic sinusitis as noted by these pediatricians in a series of 58 patients referred to us for sinusitis that failed to respond to aggressive medical management.

TABLE 1.3. *Clinical findings of acute and chronic sinusitis of children*

Clinical findings	Acute sinusitis (%)	Chronic sinusitis (%)
Symptoms		
Fever	50	20
Rhinorrhea	80	80
Cough (persistent and evening)	50	75
Pain/headache	30	30
Sore throat	20	20
Periorbital swelling	30	0
Vomiting	20	10
Allergic history	?	?
Signs		
Rhinorrhea	80	80
Temperature ≥101°F	20	0
Sinus tenderness	20	10
Otitis media	40	60
Posterior pharyngeal pus	0	10
Periorbital swelling	30	0
Laboratory		
Abnormal x-rays	100	100
Maxillary	90	90
Ethmoid	40	40
Frontal and sphenoid	10	10
Unilateral	70	10
Bilateral	30	90
Erythrocyte sedimentation rate elevation	50	10
White blood cell count elevation with an increased percentage of band form neutrophils	40	10

From ref. 4, with permission.

ACUTE SINUSITIS

Symptoms

The symptoms of acute sinusitis are frequently preceded by an upper respiratory viral illness with clear drainage. Most frequently the symptoms resolve without evidence of persistent disease (5); however, if they continue for more than 10 days one should consider sinusitis as a possibility (6–9). The presentation of the symptoms is different at different ages. Because younger children are not able to articulate their complaints well, their symptoms are not well defined; however, older children are able to localize their symptoms with much greater accuracy and present with symptoms similar to those seen in adults. Ellen Wald (5–7) indicates that sinusitis in the acute phase may manifest itself in one of two ways. The less common presentation is a "cold" that seems more severe than usual, with a fever of more than 39.0°C, purulent rhinorrhea, and facial pain. More frequently, symptoms are that of a prolonged "cold" with cough and nasal discharge persisting beyond 10 days. In this case it is not the severity of the symptoms but their persistence that calls for attention. Most viral infections last 5 to 7 days, with some not totally resolved but significantly improved by day 10 (5,7).

Symptoms other than the presenting symptoms may be discovered only by further questioning. Coughing is noted with acute sinusitis but appears to be more

TABLE 1.4. *Symptoms used to diagnose chronic sinusitis in children as reported by 45 pediatricians*

Symptoms	Frequency[a]
Purulent rhinorrhea	2.56
Cough	2.67
Fever	1.30
Headache	2.18
Sore throat	1.72
Nausea/vomiting	1.10
Bad breath	1.94

[a] 0, never; 1, seldom; 2, occasional; 3, frequent.

TABLE 1.5. *Findings associated with chronic sinusitis in 58 children*[a]

Symptoms	Number of cases	Percentage (%)
Purulent rhinorrhea	52	90
Cough	23	40
Fever	22	38
Headache	21	36
Nasal obstruction	18	31
Asthma exacerbation	15	26
Facial swelling	13	22
Sore throat	7	12
Recurrent pneumonia	7	12
Choking spells	2	3

[a] Referred for sinusitis that did not respond to aggressive medical management.

common in chronic sinusitis (4). According to Wald, the coughing must be present during the day for it to be a symptom of chronic sinusitis (5), although it may be worse at night. It is the persistent cough that frequently causes parents to seek medical evaluation for their children.

Children with acute and chronic sinusitis almost universally present with purulent nasal discharge (2,9–14), which is not characteristic in adults. Nasal airway obstruction or nasal congestion is frequently encountered but is a nonspecific symptom since there are a host of lesions that can cause either one: tonsil adenoid hypertrophy, septal deviation, allergic rhinitis, craniofacial anomaly, and thick secretions, to name a few. Parents will frequently refer to the obstruction as congestion, "being stuffy," mouth breathing, or "sinus."

Fever is infrequent even with acute sinusitis (4) and is usually associated with complicated acute sinusitis (6). The fever abates with resolution of the infection. Accurate information on the extent of fever in acute and chronic sinusitis is lacking in the literature, although it appears to be much less frequent with chronic sinusitis.

Emesis secondary to coughing, nausea, or gagging on postnasal secretions is a symptom sometimes noted, but it is infrequent in our experience. Some children frequently complain of chronic stomach ache, but it is always difficult to ascertain if this is secondary to the sinusitis or to the antibiotics used to treat the infection.

Signs

The signs vary with age. Purulent rhinorrhea is frequently noted in all age groups but is much more common in young children. The young child may present with drainage or irritation of the upper lip secondary to the purulent nasal discharge. There may be erythema of the tissue over the sinus, but in our experience this is rare and frequently is a sign of complicated sinus disease. Facial tenderness is seen more frequently in acute sinusitis but is not a frequent complaint (4,6). Examination of the nasal cavity will reveal boggy, edematous mucosa with significant obstruction. With vasoconstriction the nasal airway will open, permitting better examination. In the pediatric population, anterior rhinoscopy is usually all that can be performed regardless of the method of examination used. In acute sinusitis the purulence is usually thin and is easily suctioned from the anterior nasal vault. Occasionally one will identify purulence draining into the nasopharynx, but in our experience this is an unusual physical finding.

Otitis media is seen in both acute and chronic disease (3,15–21). The middle ear can be thought of as a highly modified paranasal sinus, and indeed, the bacteria causing infection are very similar (6,8,15,22,23). Chronic sinusitis may be associated with different sinus persistence and increased anaerobic bacteria (24–26) and no studies have been performed that attempt to correlate the bacteria found in otitis media and chronic sinusitis.

Cervical lymph adenopathy is not common in acute or chronic sinusitis.

CHRONIC SINUSITIS

Symptoms

The symptoms of chronic sinusitis are equally variable and include nasal obstruction, purulent rhinorrhea, cough, and persistent or recurrent colds. Coughing appears to be more common with chronic sinusitis (2,9,12), but it is not diagnostic. Frequent viral upper respiratory tract infections, cough variant asthma (27), bronchitis, pneumonia, and allergy may all present with cough as the chief complaint. If the cough is present during the day and night, sinusitis must be considered in the differential diagnosis (2). Night cough appears to be more common than day cough with chronic sinusitis, and sleep is frequently disrupted. Coughing in the morning, just after awakening, may be so severe that it results in emesis (1). This could be secondary to the sinopulmonary reflex or secondary to thick postnasal discharge. Holinger (27) has found sinusitis to be the second most common cause of chronic cough in children.

The constant purulent nasal discharge may manifest as postnasal drip and sore throat, but it is not frequently seen on physical examination. Chronic mouth breathing for any reason will result in sore throats in a high percentage of children (1,9,11). Pharyngitis may be frequent and is often confused with tonsillitis. Frequently chronic sinusitis is associated with acute or chronic otitis media, which is likely secondary to eustachian tube dysfunction (1).

Headaches appear to be more common in chronic sinusitis and in older children (1,9). The child may hold his/her head, display head-banging, or even find comfort by putting his/her face on a cool floor tile for pain relief. Often only in retrospect will a parent realize that such behavior may be a response to headache or facial pain. In chronic sinusitis the child may be acclimated to the pain, and the only manifestation of discomfort is irritability or mood changes.

The older patient may present with headaches as the chief complaint, and only on additional questioning will the symptoms of sinusitis be revealed. Stammberger and Wolf (28) have noted that there are three different groups of headaches:

1. Those clearly associated with sinus disease, such as inflammation, neoplasm, or barotrauma.
2. Those clearly of nonsinus origin, such as migraine, neuralgias, cervical spin disorders, hypertension, or other vascular disorders.
3. Those whose origin is not clear and which are not associated with overt sinus disease.

The typical triad for the sinus patient is nasal congestion, pathologic secretions, and headaches. The pain is usually "dull" and radiating to the top of the calvarium or bitemporal for sphenoid or posterior ethmoid disease. Pain at the glabella, inner canthus, or between the eyes suggests anterior ethmoid or frontal sinusitis. Pain over the cheeks most frequently suggests maxillary sinusitis.

A number of anatomical variations (Table 1.6) have been noted to predispose the patient to recurrent head-

TABLE 1.6. *Frequent anatomic variations predisposing to headaches and recurrent sinusitis*

Septal deviation/spurs
Agger nasi cells/enlarged or diseased
Uncinate process
  Medially bent
  Laterally bent
  Curved anteriorly ("doubled middle turbinate")
  Fractures (trauma, iatrogenic)
  Contacting turbinate
  Pneumatized
Middle turbinate
  Concha bellosa (pneumatized)
  Paradoxically bent
  Bulging into lateral nasal wall
Ethmoid bulla
  Large, filling middle meatus
  Contact areas (especially polyps)
  Anterior growth, overlapping hiatus semilunaris
  Protruding from middle meatus
Haller Cell
Combinations of all of the above

From ref. 28, with permission.

aches and sinusitis (28). These anatomical variations can best be elucidated with coronal CT scans and examination with endoscopes. A thorough examination with endoscopes requires a cooperative patient and is therefore a distinct limitation in the pediatric population.

Few would doubt the ability of sinusitis to cause pain, especially if the natural ostia are obstructed. There is the growing impression that headaches can be caused even by a relatively limited mucosal lesion or area of mucosal contact. Recent research has identified a system of neurotransmitters other than norepinephrine and acetylcholine (the neuropeptides) that may be an important factor in pain sensation. Substance P is one of these mediators controlling pain perception via unmyelinated C fibers to the cortex (28). At the site of compression, substance P can be released, causing neurogenic edema through plasma extravasation, vasodilatation, and hypersecretion. The release of substance P can be mediated through stimuli such as chemical, infectious, and thermal irritants or mechanical pressure (28). The mechanical pressure can result from inflammation, polyps, or mucosal edema secondary to anatomical defects. The release of substance P results in a vicious cycle of neurogenic edema, more release, and more edema, ultimately resulting in massive symptoms. There is some indication that capsaicin, the pungent extract of red pepper, has the ability to selectively destroy the afferent C fibers and potentially interrupt this cycle (29,30). The mediating function of substance P could therefore be treated with local administration of capsaicin without affecting other sensory structures. This might prove to be an effective medical therapeutic modality (28).

Signs

As with acute sinusitis, the mucosa is edematous and erythematous. If the ostium to the infected sinus is patent, purulence will be noted in the nose. If the ostium is occluded or if there are large polyps present, there may be little evidence of purulence in the nose. The anterior nose is frequently filled with crusts of inspissated mucus and purulence that obscure the view. Noting the location of the purulence during nasal suction will give some idea of the location of the involved sinuses (Figs. 1.1 and 1.2). If the purulence is coming from the middle meatus or medial to the middle turbinate, it likely involves the cells draining into the osteomeatal complex (5). If it is noted lateral to the middle turbinate, the posterior ethmoid cells or the sphenoid is involved. The sources of the purulence and facial tenderness are perhaps the most revealing physical findings in chronic sinusitis (5).

The adenoid pad may be hypertrophied or enlarged secondary to inflammation. This can result in nasal

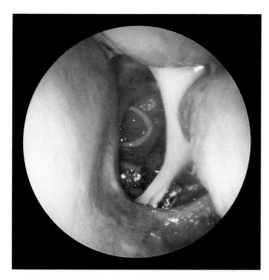

FIG. 1.1. Purulence from the superior meatus and sphenoid recess.

obstruction or fetid breath secondary to infection. The fetid breath is often dismissed by parents as poor toothbrushing or dental caries (6,9). Bad breath can also result from tonsilloliths, foreign bodies of the nasal airway, or crusting of the nasal secretions (9).

Fever is usually low if present and is not well documented in the literature of chronic sinusitis (4).

Otitis media (4) is seen more frequently (60%) in chronic otitis media. The causal relationship is not well defined but likely is secondary to eustachian tube dysfunction. Purulent secretions from the middle meatus usually course inferior to the eustachian tube while secretions from the posterior ethmoids course superiorly. On occasion the purulent secretions stagnate at the eustachian tube orifice, resulting in inflammation and direct seeding of the middle ear space.

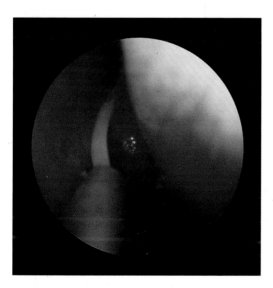

FIG. 1.2. Purulence from the superior middle meatus and the frontal recess.

REFERENCES

1. Rachelefsky GS. Sinusitis in children—diagnosis and management. *Clin Rev Allergy* 1984;2:397.
2. Rachelefsky GS, Goldberg M, Katz RM, et al. Sinus disease in children with respiratory allergy. *J Allergy Clin Immunol* 1978;61:310.
3. Hoshaw TC, Nickman NJ. Sinusitis and otitis in children. *Arch Otolaryngol* 1974;100:194.
4. Cherry JD, Dudley JP. Sinusitis. In: Cherry JD, ed. *Textbook of pediatric infectious diseases.* Philadelphia: Saunders, 1981;104.
5. Wald ER. Special series: management of pediatric infectious diseases in office practice. Acute sinusitis in children. *Pediatr Infect Dis* 1983;2:61.
6. Wald ER. Diagnosis and management of acute sinusitis. *Pediatr Ann* 1988;17:629.
7. Wald ER. The diagnosis and management of sinusitis in children. Diagnostic considerations. *Pediatr Infect Dis* 1985;4:S61.
8. Wald ER, Reilly JS, Casselbrant M, et al. Treatment of acute maxillary sinusitis in childhood: a comparative study of amoxicillin and cefaclor. *J Pediatr* 1984;104:297.
9. Wald ER, Milmoe GJ, Bowen A, Ledesma-Medina J, Salamon N, Bluestone CD. Acute maxillary sinusitis in children. *N Engl J Med* 1981;304:749.
10. Wald ER, Pang D, Milmoe GJ, Schramm VL Jr. Sinusitis and its complications in the pediatric patient. *Pediatr Clin North Am* 1981;28:777.
11. Paul D. Sinus infection and adenotonsillitis in pediatric patients. *Laryngoscope* 1981;91:997.
12. Herz G, Gfeller J. Sinusitis in paediatrics. *Chemotherapy* 1977;23:50.
13. Jaffe BF. Chronic sinusitis in children. Comments on pathogenesis and management. *Clin Pediatr (Phila)* 1974;13:944.
14. Shone GR. Maxillary sinus aspiration in children. What are the indications? *J Laryngol Otol* 1987;101:461.
15. Bluestone CD. Otitis media and sinusitis in children. Role of Branhamella catarrhalis. *Drugs* 1986;31:132.
16. Grote JJ, Kuijpers W. Middle ear effusion and sinusitis. *J Laryngol Otol* 1980;94:177.
17. Nickman NJ. Sinusitis, otitis and adenotonsillitis in children: a retrospective study. *Laryngoscope* 1978;88:117.
18. Brockman SJ. The enigma of secretory otitis media. *Trans Am Acad Ophthalmol Otolaryngol* 1972;76:1296.
19. Jaffe BF, DeBlanc CB. Sinusitis in children with cleft lip and palate. *Arch Otolaryngol* 1971;93:479.
20. Falser N, Mittermayer H, Weuta H. Antibacterial treatment of otitis and sinusitis with ciprofloxacin and penicillin V—a comparison. *Infection* 1988;16(suppl 1):S51.
21. Bluestone CD. Otitis media and sinusitis: management and when to refer to the otolaryngologist [review]. *Pediatr Infect Dis* 1987;6:100.
22. Wald ER. Epidemiology, pathophysiology and etiology of sinusitis. *Pediatr Infect Dis* 1985;4:S51.
23. Shapiro ED, Milmoe GJ, Wald ER, Rodnan JB, Bowen AD. Bacteriology of the maxillary sinuses in patients with cystic fibrosis. *J Infect Dis* 1982;146:589.
24. Brook I, Friedman EM. Intracranial complications of sinusitis in children. A sequela of periapical abscess. *Ann Otol Rhinol Laryngol* 1982;91:41.
25. Brook I. Bacteriologic features of chronic sinusitis in children. *JAMA* 1981;246:967.
26. Brook I. Frontal sinusitis [letter]. *Pediatr Infect Dis* 1984;3:284.
27. Holinger LD. Chronic cough in infants and children. *Laryngoscope* 1986;96:316.
28. Stammberger H, Wolf G. Headaches and sinus disease: the endoscopic approach. *Ann Otol Rhinol Laryngol* 1988;134:3.
29. Fitzgerald M. Capsaicin and sensory neurones—a review. *Pain* 1983;15:109.
30. Lundblad L, Brodin E, Lundberg JM, Anggard A. Effects of nasal capsaicin pretreatment and cryosurgery on sneezing reflexes, neurogenic plasma extravasation, sensory and sympathetic neurons. *Acta Otolaryngol (Stockh)* 1985;100:117.

Pediatric Sinusitis,
edited by R. P. Lusk,
Raven Press, Ltd., New York © 1992.

CHAPTER 2

Pathophysiology of Chronic Sinusitis

Rodney P. Lusk and Gerald Wolf

The causes of pediatric sinusitis are multifactorial and are not completely understood. Much of what is known is based on the pathophysiology of adult disease. Because the immunologic system and anatomy are still developing in children, there are reasons to suspect that the pathophysiology of pediatric sinusitis is different from sinusitis in adults. Nevertheless, there are compelling reasons to apply the knowledge gained through adult patients to our pediatric patients.

Siber et al. (1) estimated that 0.5% of upper respiratory infections are complicated by acute sinusitis. However, because these authors did not precisely define sinusitis, their estimate may be inaccurate. The incidence most likely falls between 0.5 and 5.0% (2). With the average adult having two to three colds per year and children six to eight (3), sinusitis is a common problem.

PATHOGENS AND IMMUNOLOGY

Hemophilus influenza and *Streptococcus* sp. as causal agents in sinus infections and complications are more common in infants than in older children (4–6). Bacteremia caused by *H. influenza, S. pneumonia,* and *Strep-pneumococcus* (84%) (7) is more common in children less than 5 years old (8,9). The older the patient, the lower the incidence of bacteremia (10).

The reasons for this may lie in the increasing ability of the growing child's body to recognize and form antibodies to the polysaccharide capsules of *H. influenza* and *Streptococcus* sp. bacteria. There is evidence that the immunologic response in young children is defective (1), possibly because of inadequate processing of the polysaccharide antigens by immature macrophages or hyporesponsive B-cell plasmocytes (8). The interaction between B-lymphocytes and subsets of T-helper cells may also be defective (8). Shapiro et al. (11) found evidence of immune deficiency in 34 of 61 children. The most common deficiencies were IgG3 and pneumococcal antigen 7. Young children have also been noted to have subclass deficiencies (12,13), which may contribute to the increased number of upper respiratory tract infections in childhood.

MUCOSAL AND CILIARY FUNCTION

The mucosa, the cilia, and the mucus blanket function as a unit. Chronic sinusitis, which may involve all or only a few of the sinuses, is the result of disease in this functional unit.

The respiratory mucosa of the nose and sinuses is not homogeneous but shows marked local differences. Mucosal biopsies have demonstrated wide variation in the histopathology of patients with polypoid hyperplastic sinusitis (14,15). The mucosal thickness and histologic makeup are dependent on physical and biological responses to metabolic, endocrine, environmental, and inflammatory factors.

The cilia are long, slender, hairlike projections extending from the ciliated mucosa. In the center of the cilia are two central microtubules surrounded by a ring of nine doublet microtubules connected by dynein arms. The cilia beat in a specific direction with a rapid forward beat and a slow return beat at about 1000 strokes per minute in the normal sinus (16).

The cilia can beat only in a fluid medium. The mucus blanket is double, with a superficial viscid fluid layer and a serous layer underneath. The thick outer layer traps bacteria and debris while the cilia beat in the thin inner layer. The cilia just touch the outer layer and, through coordinated beating, propel the thick layer along specified paths. Alterations in the mucus blan-

R. P. Lusk: Department of Otolaryngology, St. Louis Children's Hospital, St. Louis, Missouri 63110.

G. Wolf: University HNO-Clinic, A-8010 Graz, Austria.

ket, as in asthma and cystic fibrosis, impair ciliary motility and are associated with recurrent infections of the upper respiratory tract.

There is a close association between ciliary function and the health of the sinus. Messerklinger (17) noted that pressure between two mucosal surfaces, as the result of inflammation, edema, or anatomical variations, resulted in inhibited ciliary function and secondary stasis of secretions. These secretions can become secondarily infected from bacteria residing in the nose and result in clinical sinusitis.

It is well known that abnormal cilia are associated with chronic sinusitis (18–24). The most common abnormality is in the dynein arms (18). Some investigators feel that there is still some motility in these defective cilia, but in any case, chronic sinusitis is not necessarily associated with abnormal ciliary ultrastructure (25).

Toxins associated with bacterial and viral infections can also inhibit ciliary function (26). This was recognized very early when King (27) noted that oil was not being extruded from the maxillary sinuses of patients with acute infections. Mygind et al. (28) noted that bacterial infections are associated with fewer ciliated cells but that there seems to be a longer-lasting loss of ciliated cells with viral infections. Temporarily acquired ciliary defects have been observed in nasal mucosa of children with acute viral upper respiratory infections. Wilson et al. (26) noted that ciliary clearance, as measured by the saccharin method, was prolonged in infected patients and that the beat frequency was slower (12.3 Hz) in infected patients than in normal controls (14.3 Hz). They felt that inhibited function was secondary to toxins produced by the inflammatory response and not caused by the bacteria themselves.

An overall temporal view of the nonspecific inflammatory responses of the mucosa is not yet available. It is suspected that an intermediate stage of inflammation results in stasis of blood flow, tissue damage, edema, and lymphatic swelling, followed by an increase and change in character of the secretions, with a reduction in ciliary transport. Anatomical deformity can narrow the opening of any sinus and inhibit the ciliary function.

Some investigators have tried to improve ciliary function pharmacokinetically, with varying success. ATP (29), terbutaline aerosol (a β-adrenergic stimulant) (30), and adenosine triphosphate (31) have been found in clinical trials to enhance cilia motility, but their use has not gained wide acceptance.

OBSTRUCTION

At the heart of our current understanding of chronic sinusitis is the idea that obstruction in the osteomeatal complex, or openings of the sinuses, results in stasis of secretions and recurrent sinus disease (2,32–38). The obstruction may be anatomical or mucosal. Gas exchange in an obstructed sinus may be impaired, creating an anaerobic environment that favors growth of anaerobic bacteria (39). When the ostia become obstructed, a vicious cycle of ciliary dysfunction, retention of secretions, obstruction of lymphatic drainage, edema, and mucosal hyperplasia develops and may at some point become irreversible disease. It has become apparent, however, that even extensive mucosal disease is potentially reversible and at surgery neither visualization nor biopsy enables us to predict whether the inflamed mucosa will become normal (although structures such as polyps and retention cysts seem to have little potential for recovery) (40).

The theory of obstruction causing sinusitis is not new. Hajek (41) in 1929 noted that obstruction and edema of the mucosa in the middle meatus were central to the cause of recurrent frontal sinusitis. Zuckerkandl (42) also recognized the importance of anatomical variations in the middle meatus as a cause of recurrent sinusitis. Rice and Schaefer (43) noted that in 1916 J. Parsons Schaeffer (44) stated that ''the maxillary sinus is often a cesspool for infectious material from the sinus frontalis and certain of the anterior group of the cellulae ethmoidales.'' The preantibiotic physicians understood the importance of these drainage sites; that knowledge was lost with the advent of antibiotics and rediscovered when better visualization was possible through telescopes (17,32,38,45), tomography, and CT scans (17,35,46) and through the work of Messerklinger (17) and Wigand et al. (47). Although it is clear that osteomeatal complex obstruction in children is a factor, it is not clear whether the obstruction is *the* primary cause of chronic or recurrent sinusitis in children.

ANATOMY

The anatomy of children's sinuses is similar to that in adults, but, especially in younger children, the structures are so much smaller that they present various problems. The smallness and the increased incidence of upper respiratory tract infections in young children may increase the chance of obstruction and predispose these patients for recurrent sinus infections. If the mucosal disease is localized, surgical intervention is particularly useful. If, on the other hand, the mucosal disease is more systemic, surgical intervention is potentially less successful because the diseased mucosa must reline the surgical defect.

There are a number of potential sites for obstruction, which may occur at the opening of the sinus or at more distal sites of drainage, such as the osteomeatal complex.

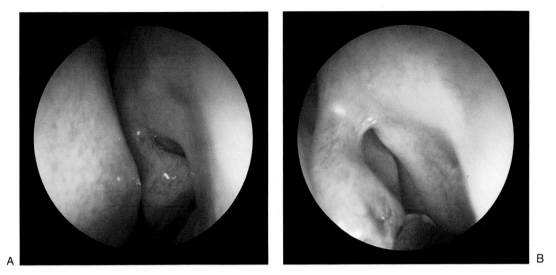

FIG. 2.1. **A:** Paradoxical left middle turbinate with a prominent agger nasi cell. **B:** View of the uncinate process with retraction of the paradoxical middle turbinate.

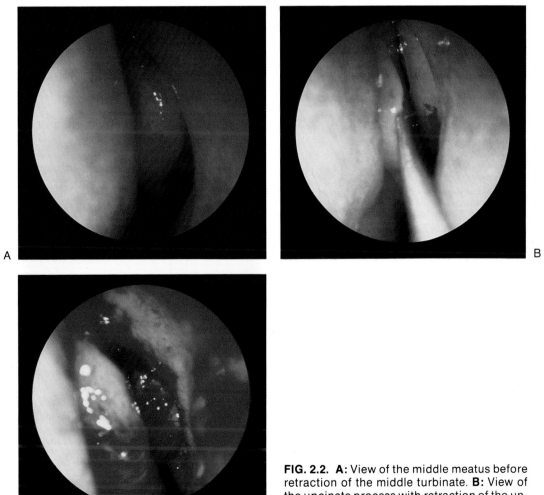

FIG. 2.2. **A:** View of the middle meatus before retraction of the middle turbinate. **B:** View of the uncinate process with retraction of the uncinate process. **C:** View of the ethmoid bulla after the uncinate process has been removed.

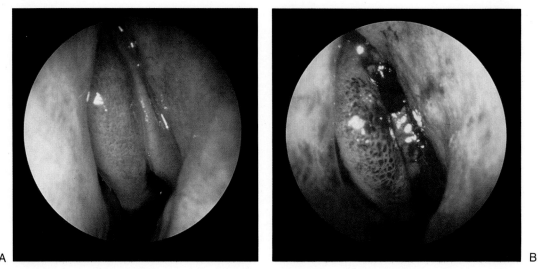

FIG. 2.3. A: Markedly enlarged uncinate process; sometimes called a doubled middle turbinate. **B:** View of the ethmoid bulla after the uncinate process has been removed.

The infundibulum is a space bordered by the uncinate process medially and the lamina papyracea laterally. Into it drain the frontal sinus (superiorly), the anterior ethmoid sinuses, and the maxillary sinus (inferiorly and posteriorly). The infundibulum communicates with the middle meatus through the hiatus semilunaris, which is the space between the posterior border of the uncinate process and the anterior face of the ethmoid bulla. This space and the surrounding area are known as the osteomeatal complex. It is felt to hold the key to the cure of recurrent and chronic sinusitis (32,33,37,48–53).

The agger nasi cells can be enlarged or diseased and cause obstruction of the frontal recess or osteomeatal complex. The infections may spread to the frontal or

ethmoid sinuses or vice versa. Endoscopically, the agger nasi cell looks like an expansion from the lateral nasal wall at the incision of the middle turbinate (Fig. 2.1A). This is a difficult area to visualize, and disease may be noted only on coronal CT scans. Agger nasi cell enlargement is usually, but not always, bilateral.

The uncinate process forms the anterior wall of the osteomeatal complex. It may be deflected medially or laterally and cause mucosal contact, which can interrupt normal mucociliary clearance. A variety of shapes of the uncinate process can predispose a patient to developing sinusitis (Figs. 2.1–2.4). The process may be large and curve out like the brim of a hat (Fig. 2.3), a condition called the "doubled middle turbinate" (36), or it may be quite small and rudimentary, as in a hy-

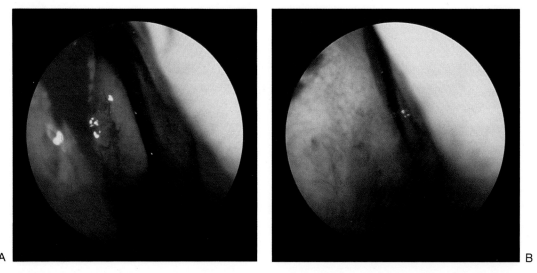

FIG. 2.4. A: Uncinate process located far forward of the middle turbinate. **B:** View of the ethmoid bulla after the uncinate process has been removed. Note the position of the middle turbinate adjacent to the ethmoid bulla.

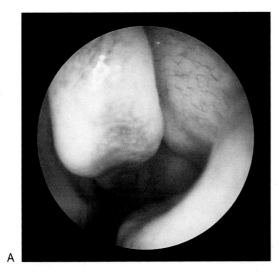
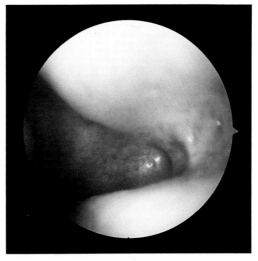

A   B

FIG. 2.5. A: View of hypoplastic maxillary sinus through the middle meatus. Superior and lateral is the floor of the orbit. It is commonly thought that the uncinate process is absent; however, with careful inspection this usually is discovered not to be the case. **B:** View of the occluded maxillary ostium. Just superior to this is a thin rudimentary uncinate process.

poplastic maxillary sinus (Fig. 2.5), or it may be pneumatized (49) and obstruct the infundibulum. The uncinate process can also be deformed by a pneumatized or paradoxical middle turbinate, which can cause minor or severe compression of the delicate structures in the area of the infundibulum (Fig. 2.1). Areas of extensive mucosal contact and obstruction of the middle meatus can be caused by a concha bullosa. These deformities may predispose the patient to sinusitis or, in the older patient, be manifest only as a headache.

The ethmoid bulla can be significantly pneumatized and obstruct the middle meatus. It can extend medially onto the middle turbinate, anteriorly into the infundibulum, or anteriorly and laterally into the maxillary

sinus ostium. Each of these areas can create obstruction severe enough to cause stasis of secretions and subsequent sinusitis.

There is considerable variability in the size and shape of the maxillary sinus ostium. Its occlusion may result in recurrent or chronic maxillary sinusitis. The ostium is located in the posterior half of the hiatus semilunaris in 94% of adult patients (54), and in our experience, the location is much the same in children. The size of the ostium in adults ranges from 2 to 7 mm (55), but reliable measurements have not been published for children. The shape of the ostium varies from round to slitlike to triangular, but the importance of

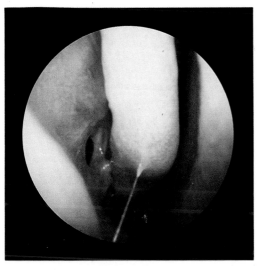

FIG. 2.6. Accessory ostium of the maxillary sinus, inferior to the uncinate process.

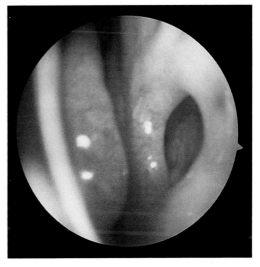

FIG. 2.7. Accessory ostium of the uncinate process; the accessory ostium allows one to look directly into the infundibulum.

the shape is not known. The ostium may also be narrowed by a Haller cell (Fig. 2.4), increasing the chance of functional obstruction.

In adults, Draf (55) noted that 13% of patients have an accessory ostium. One percent of the accessory ostia are larger than the natural ostia, and 1 to 2% are multiple ostia. The etiology of accessory ostia is not known, but it is commonly thought to be secondary to chronic or recurrent inflammation. This has not been proved, however. Accessory ostia occur in children as well as adults (Figs. 2.6 and 2.7) and can occur in patients without evidence of acute inflammation at the time of the surgical procedure.

Other etiologies of chronic sinusitis are elaborated on in the following chapters. A more detailed discussion of the association between tonsil and adenoid hypertrophy and infections is presented in Chapter 10 (pp. 77–79).

REFERENCES

1. Siber GRT, Schur PH, Aisenberg AC. Correlation between serum IgG-2 concentrations and the antibody response to bacterial polysaccharide antigens. *N Engl J Med* 1980;303:178–182.
2. Wald ER. Epidemiology, pathophysiology and etiology of sinusitis. *Pediatr Infect Dis* 1985;4:S51–S54.
3. Gwaltney JM Jr, Sydnor AJ Jr, Sande MA. Etiology and antimicrobial treatment of acute sinusitis. *Ann Otol Rhinol Laryngol [Suppl]* 1981;90:68–71.
4. Rubinstein JB, Handler SD. Orbital and periorbital cellulitis in children. *Head Neck Surg* 1982;5:15–21.
5. Revonta M, Suonpaa J. Diagnosis of subacute maxillary sinusitis in children. *J Laryngol Otol* 1981;95:133–140.
6. Ylikoski J, Savolainen S, Jousimies-Somer H. The bacteriology of acute maxillary sinusitis. *ORL J Otorhinolaryngol Relat Spec* 1989;51:175–181.
7. Decreton SJ, Clement PA. Comparative study of standard x-ray of the maxillary sinus and sinuscopy in children. *Rhinology* 1981;19:155–159.
8. Weiss A, Friendly D, Eglin K, Chang M, Gold B. Bacterial periorbital and orbital cellulitis in childhood. *Ophthalmology* 1983;90:195–203.
9. Schramm VL Jr, Myers EN, Kennerdell JS. Orbital complications of acute sinusitis: evaluation, management, and outcome. *OTOL AAOO* 1978;86:221–230.
10. Schramm VL Jr, Carter HD, Kennerdell JS. Evaluation of orbital cellulitis and results of treatment. *Laryngoscope* 1982; 92:732–738.
11. Shapiro GG, Virant FS, Furukawa CT, Pierson WE, Bierman CW. Immunologic defects in patients with refractory sinusitis. *Pediatrics* 1991;87:311–316.
12. Morell A, Skvaril F, Hitzig WH. IgG subclasses: development of the serum concentrations in "normal" infants and children. *J Pediatr* 1972;80:960–964.
13. Shur PH, Rosen F, Norman ME. Immunoglobulin subclasses in normal children. *Pediatr Res* 1979;13:181–183.
14. Hosemann W, Wigand ME, Fehle R, Sebastian J, Diepgen DL. Results of endonasal ethmoid bone operations in diffuse hyperplastic chronic paranasal sinusitis. [Ergebnisse endonasaler Siebbein-Operationen bei diffuser hyperplastischer Sinusitis paranasalis chronica.] *HNO* 1988;36:54–59.
15. Hosemann WG. Endoscopically controlled paranasal sinus operations [in German]. *Dtsch Krankenpflegezeitschrift* 1990; 43:509–513.
16. Reimer A, von Mecklenburg C, Toremalm NG. The mucociliary activity of the upper respiratory tract. III: A functional and morphological study of human and animal material with special reference to maxillary sinus disease. *Acta Otolaryngol [Suppl] (Stockh)* 1978;355:3–20.
17. Messerklinger W. *Endoscopy of the nose.* Baltimore: Urban & Schwarzenberg, 1978.
18. Eavey RD, Nadol JB Jr, Holmes LB, Laird NM, Lapey A, Joseph MP. Kartagener's syndrome. A blinded, controlled study of cilia ultrastructure. *Arch Otolaryngol Head Neck Surg* 1986;112:646–650.
19. Karja J, Nuutinen J. Immotile cilia syndrome in children. *Int J Pediatr Otorhinolaryngol* 1983;5:275–279.
20. Mygind N, Pedersen M. Nose-, sinus- and ear-symptoms in 27 patients with primary ciliary dyskinesia. *Eur J Respir Dis [Suppl]* 1983;127:96–101.
21. Pedersen M, Mygind N. Rhinitis, sinusitis and otitis media in Kartagener's syndrome (primary ciliary dyskinesia). *Clin Otolaryngol* 1982;7:373–380.
22. Yarnal JF, Golish JA, Ahmad M, Tomashefski JF. The immotile cilia syndrome: explanation for many a clinical mystery. *Postgrad Med* 1982;71:195–197,200–202.
23. Imbrie JD. Kartagener's syndrome: a genetic defect affecting the function of cilia. *Am J Otolaryngol* 1981;2:215–222.
24. Lupin AJ, Misko GJ. Kartagener syndrome with abnormalities of cilia. *J Otolaryngol* 1978;7:95–102.
25. Fontolliet C, Terrier G. Abnormalities of cilia and chronic sinusitis. *Rhinology* 1987;25:57–62.
26. Wilson R, Sykes DA, Currie D, Cole PJ. Beat frequency of cilia from sites of purulent infection. *Thorax* 1986;41:453–458.
27. King E. A clinical study of the functioning of the maxillary sinus mucosa. *Ann Otol Rhinol Laryngol* 1935;44:480–482.
28. Mygind N, Pedersen M, Nielsen MH. Primary and secondary ciliary dyskinesia. *Acta Otolaryngol (Stockh)* 1983;95:688–694.
29. Jakubíková J, Kapellerová A, Klaèansky I. Activation of damaged nasal mucociliary function in children [in Czechoslovakian]. *Cesk Otolaryngol* 1989;38:45–47.
30. Ohashi Y, Nakai Y, Zushi K, et al. Enhancement of ciliary action by a beta-adrenergic stimulant. *Acta Otolaryngol [Suppl] (Stockh)* 1983;397:49–59.
31. Nuutinen J. Activation of the impaired nasal mucociliary transport in children: preliminary report. *Int J Pediatr Otorhinolaryngol* 1985;10:47–52.
32. Kennedy DW, Zinreich SJ, Shaalan H, Kuhn F, Naclerio R, Loch E. Endoscopic middle meatal antrostomy: theory, technique, and patency. *Laryngoscope* 1987;97:1–9.
33. Stammberger H. Endoscopic endonasal surgery—concepts in treatment of recurring rhinosinusitis. Part II. Surgical technique. *Otolaryngol Head Neck Surg* 1986;94:147–156.
34. Eichel B. Ethmoiditis. Pathophysiology and medical management. *Otolaryngol Clin North Am* 1985;18:43–53.
35. Kennedy DW, Zinreich SJ, Rosenbaum AE, Johns ME. Functional endoscopic sinus surgery. Theory and diagnostic evaluation. *Arch Otolaryngol* 1985;111:576–582.
36. Stammberger H, Wolf G. Headaches and sinus disease: the endoscopic approach. *Ann Otol Rhinol Laryngol* 1988;134:3–23.
37. Stammberger H. Nasal and paranasal sinus endoscopy. A diagnostic and surgical approach to recurrent sinusitis. *Endoscopy* 1986;18:213–218.
38. Stammberger H. Endoscopic endonasal surgery—concepts in treatment of recurring rhinosinusitis. Part I. Anatomic and pathophysiologic considerations. *Otolaryngol Head Neck Surg* 1986;94:143–147.
39. Drettner B. Pathophysiology of paranasal sinuses with clinical implications. *Clin Otolaryngol* 1980;5:272–284.
40. Wigand ME. *Endoscopic surgery of the paranasal sinuses and anterior skull base.* New York: Thieme Medical Publishers, 1990.
41. Hajek M. *Pathology and treatment of the inflammatory diseases of the nasal accessory sinuses.* St. Louis: Mosby, 1926.
42. Zuckerkandl E. *Pathology and treatment of the inflammatory diseases of the nasal accessory sinuses.* St Louis: Mosby, 1926;99.
43. Rice DH, Schaefer SD. *Endoscopic paranasal sinus surgery.* New York: Raven Press, 1988.

44. Schaeffer J. The genesis, development and adult anatomy of the nasofrontal region in man. *Am J Anat* 1916;20:125–146.
45. Kennedy DW, Zinreich SJ, Kumar AJ, Rosenbaum AE, Johns ME. Physiologic mucosal changes within the nose and ethmoid sinus: imaging of the nasal cycle by MRI. *Laryngoscope* 1988;98:928–933.
46. Stammberger H. Personal endoscopic operative technique for the lateral nasal wall—an endoscopic surgery concept in the treatment of inflammatory diseases of the paranasal sinuses. [Unsere endoskopische Operationstechnik der lateralen Nasenwand—ein endoskopisch-chirurgisches Konzept zur Behandlung entzundlicher Nasennebenhohlenerkrankungen.] *Laryngol Rhinol Otol (Stuttg)* 1985;64:559–566.
47. Wigand ME, Steiner W, Jaumann MP. Endonasal sinus surgery with endoscopical control: from radical operation to rehabilitation of the mucosa. *Endoscopy* 1978;10:255–260.
48. Stammberger H, Posawetz W. Functional endoscopic sinus surgery. Concept, indications and results of the Messerklinger technique. *Eur Arch Oto-rhino-laryngol* 1990;247:63–76.
49. Zinreich SJ, Kennedy DW, Rosenbaum AE, Gayler BW, Kumar AJ. Paranasal sinuses: CT imaging requirements for endoscopic surgery. *Radiology* 1987;163:769–775.
50. Kennedy DW. Serious misconceptions regarding functional endoscopic sinus surgery [letter]. *Laryngoscope* 1986;96:1170–1171.
51. Kennedy DW, Kennedy EM. Endoscopic sinus surgery. *AORN J* 1985;42:932–934.
52. Lusk RP, Muntz HR. Endoscopic sinus surgery in children with chronic sinusitis—a pilot study. *Laryngoscope* 1990;100:654–658.
53. Lusk RP, Polmar SH, Muntz HR. Endoscopic ethmoidectomy and maxillary antrostomy in immunodeficient patients. *Arch Otolaryngol Head Neck Surg* 1991;117:60–63.
54. Lang J. *Clinical anatomy of the nose, nasal cavity and paranasal sinuses.* New York: Thieme Medical Publishers, 1989;50–53.
55. Draf W. *Endoscopy of the paranasal sinuses.* New York: Springer-Verlag, 1983.

Pediatric Sinusitis,
edited by R. P. Lusk,
Raven Press, Ltd., New York © 1992.

CHAPTER 3

Imaging of Sinusitis in Infants and Children

William H. McAlister, Thomas E. Herman, and Franz J. Wippold II

Controversy surrounds the diagnosis of sinusitis in infants and children. Some authors have claimed that only radiographically clear sinuses are normal while others state that clouding is seen from crying, redundant normal mucosa, upper respiratory infections, and allergies. Adding to the difficulty are the often nonspecific clinical findings of sinusitis. Realizing these issues, the imaging techniques for sinusitis in the pediatric population are reviewed.

PLAIN RADIOGRAPHS

Plain radiographs of the sinuses are less expensive, widely available, and usually will suffice in acute or uncomplicated sinusitis (1). The standard projections

W. H. McAlister, T. E. Herman, and F. J. Wippold II: Mallinckrodt Institute of Radiology, Washington University School of Medicine, St. Louis, Missouri 63110.

for the paranasal sinuses have been used for many years and include Waters (2) (Fig. 3.1), Caldwell (3) (Fig. 3.2), lateral (Fig. 3.3), and basal view or submentovertex (Fig. 3.4). The Waters projection is primarily used for the maxillary sinuses, the Caldwell for the ethmoid and frontals, and the lateral and basal views for the sphenoid sinuses, although each view provides additional information about the other sinuses. A Waters view with the head turned on its side in a decubitus position may make the detection of air–fluid levels easier to detect in children with small sinuses (4,5). An open mouth Waters will show a portion of the sphenoid sinuses in older children. The lateral view is of limited value in children under the age of 3 to 4 years due to limited development of the sphenoid sinuses except for the evaluation of adenoidal enlargement (Fig. 3.5). Nasal secretions and the turbinates limit the usefulness of the basal view in the evaluation of the ethmoid sinuses. In infants and young children, we take the radiographs in the supine position while

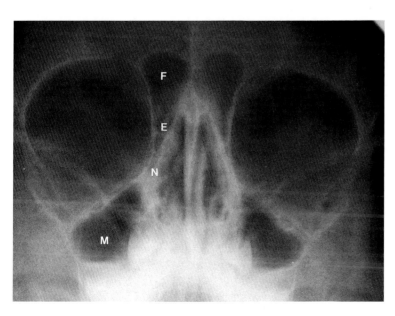

FIG. 3.1. Waters projection. The maxillary (M), anterior ethmoids (E), and frontal (F) sinuses are seen and labeled on the right. N, nasal bone.

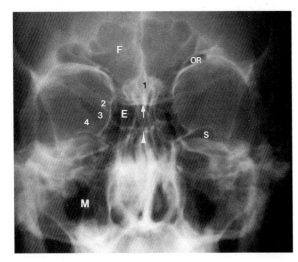

FIG. 3.2. Caldwell projeciton. The frontal (F), ethmoids (E), and maxillary (M) sinuses are shown. The sphenoid (S) sinuses have extended into the greater wing of the sphenoid. There is pneumatization of the orbital roof (OR). *Arrow*, sphenoid body; 1, crista galli; 2, lesser wing of the sphenoid; 3, superior orbital fissure; 4, greater wing of the spheniod. *Arrowhead*, sellar floor.

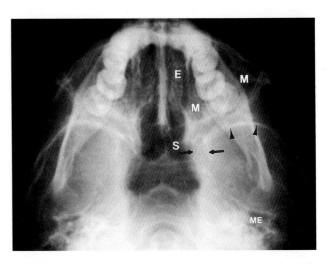

FIG. 3.4. Submentovertex projection showing the ethmoids (E), sphenoid (S), and maxillary (M) sinuses. ME, middle ear; *arrowheads*, greater wings of the sphenoid; *arrows*, pterygoid plates.

in slightly older children the radiographs are taken with the patient erect. Under the age of 6 years, we use the rule of 5's for the Waters projections (6); that is, there was less beam angulation in the younger patients (6). The beam angle increased by 5 degrees per year to 30 degrees; that is, it was zero at birth and 30 degrees at

age 6. The beam angulations were not precise due to lack of patient cooperation. At birth aerated ethmoid cells and maxillary sinuses are seen. The ethmoid sinuses increase in size until adulthood. Hypoplasia and aplasia of the ethmoids are uncommon (7). The ethmoid sinuses are divided into anterior and posterior cell groups. Some authors call a portion of the anterior cells the middle cells. The maxillary sinuses are ovoid

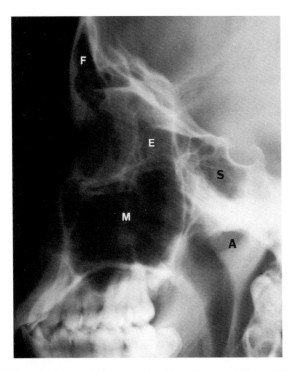

FIG. 3.3. Lateral sinus projection. The maxillary (M) sinuses are superimposed. The frontal (F), ethmoids (E), and sphenoid (S) sinuses are seen. A, adenoids.

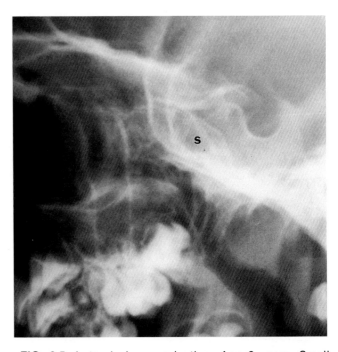

FIG. 3.5. Lateral sinus projection. Age 3 years. Small sphenoid sinuses (S) are seen. Unless the sphenoid sinus is well developed, it is difficult to evaluate on the lateral projection. One sphenoid sinus on the right was opacified while the other on the left was normal on a CT examination.

and measure less than 5 mm at birth and pneumatization occurs about 2 mm/year and then slows at age 9. They increase in size until adulthood. The mean size of the maxillary sinuses is 8 mm at ages 0 to 2, 13 mm at ages 3 to 6, 19 mm at ages 7 to 11, and 23 mm at age 12 and older (8,9). The maxillary sinuses may have asymmetric development with unilateral hypoplasia being found in 9% of children (10). The maxillary sinuses grow laterally under the orbits and inferiorly near the maxillary alveolar ridge. The sphenoid sinus develops from the right and the left posterior ethmoids at the age of 1 to 2 years but the nasal portion of the sinus does not extend to the sphenoid bone until 3 or 4 years of age. The sphenoid sinuses vary considerably in size and shape (11). The cells are usually divided by partial septa. The aerated sinuses may extend into the greater wings of the sphenoid or pterygoid plates. The sphenoid is the first sinus to achieve full development. Frontal sinuses appear at 5 to 7 years of age and also vary in size and symmetry. The bony margins are usually scalloped when the sinuses are more developed. In patients with normally developed frontal sinuses, the apparent radiographic transparency of the orbits is that of the frontal sinuses. Pneumatization may extend into the orbital roof.

Complicating factors in the plain film evaluation of the paranasal sinuses are the variability in size, shape, and pneumatization of the sinuses from birth to adolescence. The interpretations of sinus plain films in infants and young children may be difficult and the significance of sinus clouding uncertain. A number of series have reported sinus opacification without clinical sinusitis in the pediatric population, especially in infants and younger children. Some studies of normal children include those by Maresh (8) in which the percentage of sinus opacification was 60% in subjects less than 1 year, 30% in those under 5 years, and 15% in those over 12 years; Shopfner and Rossi (12) and Odita et al. (9) found sinus opacification in 57% and 54%, respectively. In one study the percentage of children under the age of 2 with sinus clouding was 76% while above that age it was 20 to 30%. Uhari found that 31% of (unselected) Finnish school children had maxillary sinus clouding (13). The lowest figure of sinus clouding in normal children was found by Kovatch to be 7% and excluded all patients who had a history of respiratory infections within the past month (14). Some feel that sinuses are normal only when they are clear. Others interpret mucous membrane thickening as abnormal if it is greater than 3 or even 4 mm (15).

The causes of sinus clouding in the absence of clinical sinus disease may be multiple, for example, obstruction of the sinus ostia with accumulation of secretion within the sinuses, swelling of the mucosa within the sinus, and small sinuses. A number of studies have shown the sinuses to be opacified in 50 to 75% of asthmatics and virtually 100% of those with cystic fibrosis (16). Allergic children have more opacification of their sinuses. The sinus mucosal abnormalities found on biopsy in patients with asthma are similar to that found in the bronchial mucosa of asthmatics (17). Therefore the sinus changes in asthmatics and those with respiratory allergies and cystic fibrosis may represent noninfectious inflammation. However, obstruction of sinus drainage and increased secretions may result in superimposed bacterial sinusitis.

Interestingly, one investigator obtained fluid from the maxillary sinuses in 39% of patients who had clinical symptoms of sinusitis but normal sinus radiographs (18). This chance of obtaining fluid fell to 15% in patients over 12 years of age. Conversely, aspiration of opacified sinuses may not yield fluid or bacteria.

Predicting multiple sinus involvement based on the plain radiographic findings of a single sinus cannot be done accurately (19). In a study of children with recurrent sinusitis, ethmoid disease was shown to be present on coronal CT in 25% of those patients with normal maxillary sinuses on a Waters projection. When the maxillary sinuses were abnormal on the Waters projections, the ethmoid sinuses were normal on coronal CT in 25% (19). Plain paranasal sinus radiographs are not adequate in determining the extent of residual involvement in recurrent sinusitis needing endoscopic surgical procedures for treatment or in complicated sinusitis with orbital cellulitis or subdural empyema.

COMPUTED TOMOGRAPHY

The anatomic detail of the sinuses supplied by the use of computed tomography (CT) has been an important factor in the growth of *functional endoscopic sinus surgery* (FES) (20). The surgeon can individualize therapy for each patient based on clinical and CT findings (21). Computed tomography of the sinuses can be accomplished using a variety of techniques (22,23). It is likely that three-dimensional (3-D) CT imaging will be used preoperatively more frequently. In addition, exciting work to provide constant 3-D CT intraoperative monitoring of surgical equipment location in the nasal cavity and sinuses is undergoing trials. Therefore the relationship of the endoscope to the orbit, the cribiform plate, and so on could be determined during the actual surgical procedure. The primary roles of coronal sinus CT are to determine the underlying cause of the sinus disease by the detailed anatomy provided and to detect the complications of sinusitis.

We use coronal scans with the patient prone and neck extended. Infants and younger children are placed supine with neck extended in a ''hanging head'' position. The scout lateral scan is used as a guide for the gantry angle in achieving the coronal plane. We use slice thicknesses of 4 mm at 3-mm intervals. The slice overlap aids in sagittal reformatting. The reformatted images can be magnified to allow anatomic direct measurements on the images. Measurements useful to some endoscopic surgeons can be made from the inferior nasal spine to three points: the superior portion of the anterior ethmoids, the midportion of the ethmoids, and the sphenoid sinus. The images are enlarged to fill the screen. Images are photographed at a window setting of 2000 H.U. with a center at 0 H.U. Some authors use a lower center or different slice thickness. Infants and younger children are sedated with intravenous nembutal and monitored by nurses familiar with the routine of the department. A variety

of other sedation practices such as oral chloral hydrate and intramuscular nembutal can be used. Pulse oximeters are used routinely in sedated patients. CO_2 monitors are also valuable. Occasionally iodine-containing contrast is given intravenously to improve soft tissue differentiation. Mucosa will enhance and can be separated from abscesses or retained sinus secretions.

CT of the paranasal sinuses beautifully demonstrates the ethmoid and sphenoid air cells and the normal or diseased osteomeatal complex (Figs. 3.6 and 3.7) without superimposed bone and air. The anatomic detail and delineation of disease in the ethmoids and osteomeatal complex by plain radiographs are limited. The normal mucosa is too thin to identify. The thin bony structures in the sinonasal region are well shown (24).

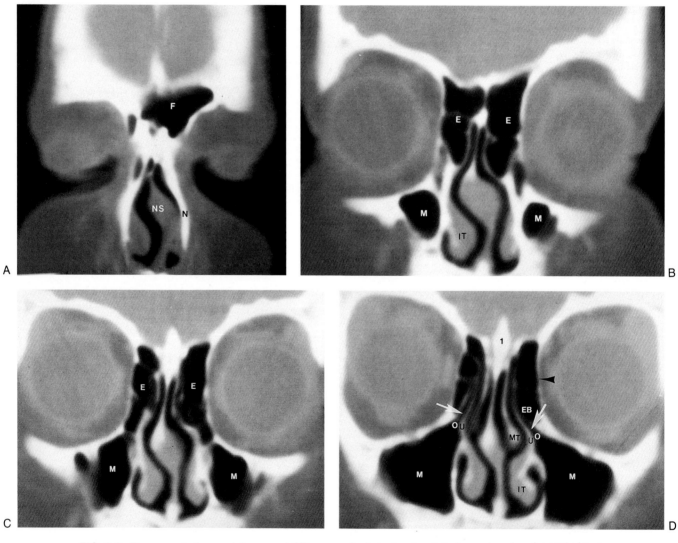

FIG. 3.6. Representative serial coronal CT scans. **A:** Anterior frontal sinus showing frontal sinus (F), nasal bone (N), and nasal septum (NS). **B:** The anterior ethmoid (E) and maxillary (M) sinuses and inferior turbinates (IT) are seen. **C, D:** At a slightly more posterior plane of the anterior ethmoids (E) and maxillary (M) sinuses the following are identified: ethmoid bulla (EB), infundibulum (*arrows*), ostea of the maxillary sinuses (O), inferior (IT) and middle (MT) turbinates, lamina papyracea (*arrowhead*), uncinate process (U), and crista galli (1). The ethmoid bulla is bounded laterally by the lamina papyracea, medially by the middle meatus, inferiorly by the infundibulum, and posteriorly by the sinus lateralis.

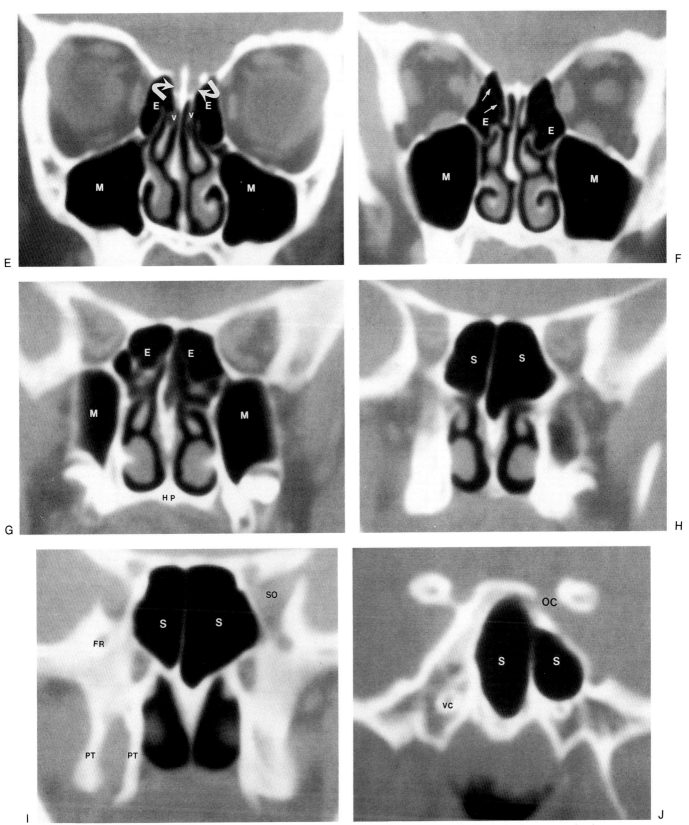

FIG. 3.6. (*Continued*) **E, F:** Middle ethmoid (E) and maxillary (M) sinuses are shown, as is the ground lamella (*arrows*) that represents the attachment of the middle turbinate to the lamina papyracea. *Curved arrows*, thin part of ethmoidal roof built by the lateral lamella of the cribriform plate; V, vertical attachment of middle turbinate to the cribriform plate. **G:** Posterior ethmoids (E) and maxillary (M) sinuses. HP, hard palate. **H–J:** The sphenoid sinus (S) is shown divided by a septum. The superior orbital fissure (SO) and the pterygoid plates (PT) are seen. OC, optic canal; VC, vidian canal; FR, foramen rotundum.

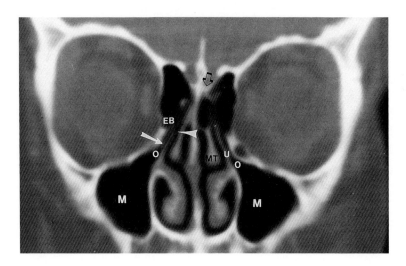

FIG. 3.7. Normal coronal sinus CT scan. A normal osteomeatal complex is seen. U, uncinate process; *arrow*, infundibulum; M, maxillary sinus; EB, ethmoid bulla; 2, middle turbinate; *arrowhead*, middle meatus; *open arrow*, cribriform plate.

The ethmoid sinuses are composed of 3 to 18 cells that drain into both adjacent cells and the nasal cavity. The cells are smaller and more numerous anteriorly. Coronal CT allows the ethmoid cells to be imaged separately (25). The ethmoid air cells are bounded laterally by the lamina papyracea, medially by the perpendicular plate or middle and superior turbinates, superiorly by the orbital plate of the frontal bone, and inferiorly by the inferior turbinate. Coronal CT is preferred although axial CT with coronal reformations is satisfactory for those who are unable to be positioned for direct coronal studies. The role of a limited CT screening examination compared to a standard coronal sinus CT is unclear. Dental amalgam can produce artifacts. Line diagrams are useful in describing the abnormalities found on coronal CT and in transmitting that information to surgeons (26).

The osteomeatal complex is a critically important area in the development of sinusitis because its narrow channel drains all but the posterior ethmoid and sphenoid sinuses (Figs. 3.6 and 3.7). The osteomeatal unit includes the ethmoid bulla, hiatus semilunaris, middle turbinate, maxillary sinus ostium and infundibulum, and the frontal recess (22,23,27). The ethmoid bulla is an air cell of variable size and shape. It is bordered laterally by the lamina papyracea, inferomedially by the infundibulum and the hiatus semilunaris, and superoposteriorly by the sinus lateralis or basal lamella. The infundibulum is a curved space located between the ethmoid bulla posteriorly and the uncinate process anteriorly. It is bounded laterally by the orbit, superiorly by frontal recess, and is open medially to the nose through a slit known as the hiatus semilunaris. The hiatus semilunaris opens into the middle meatus and is just lateral to the middle turbinate.

The middle turbinate, located inferomedial to the anterior ethmoid air cells, has bony attachments to the cribriform plate superiorly and to the lamina papyracea laterally at the level of the basal lamella. The basal lamella is obliquely oriented. If a space forms anterior to the lamella and posterior to the ethmoid bulla, it is called the sinus lateralis and may arch superiorly over

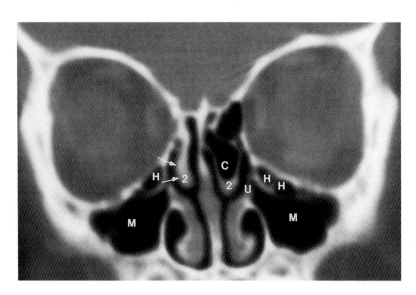

FIG. 3.8. Concha bullosa (C) and Haller cells (H) shown on coronal CT scans. U, uncinate process; 2, middle turbinate; *arrows*, paradoxic middle turbinate.

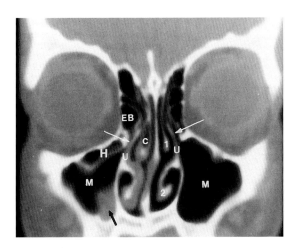

FIG. 3.9. Haller cells. Coronal CT scan showing Haller cells (H) on right, concha bullosa (C), mucous membrane thickening (*arrow*) in the right maxillary sinuses, and septal deviation. 2, middle turbinate; 1, inferior turbinate; U, uncinate process; EB, ethmoid bulla; *white arrows*, infundibulum. Note narrowing of infundibulum by Haller cells on the right.

the ethmoid bulla. The frontal recess drains the frontal sinus.

Contact between opposing mucosal surfaces produces disruption of the normal mucociliary clearance. In patients with recurrent sinusitis, the most frequent site of this mechanically induced mucociliary dysfunction is in the osteomeatal complex. Also, mucociliary dysfunction can occur at the ostia of the maxillary, ethmoid, and frontal sinuses (28). Impaired drainage through the osteomeatal complex induced by changes in the anterior ethmoids can lead to chronic maxillary and frontal sinusitis. Disease of the osteo-

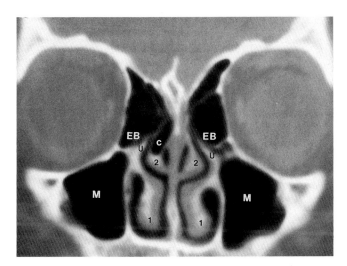

FIG. 3.10. Ethmoid bulla. Coronal CT scan shows prominent ethmoid bullae (EB). M, maxillary sinus; U, uncinate process; C, concha bullosa; 2, middle turbinate; 1, inferior turbinate.

meatal complex, however, does not necessarily result in frontal sinus disease. The frontal sinus may drain into a recess that is separate from the infundibulum and therefore be spared (29). The sphenoid drains into the sphenoid recess and the posterior ethmoidal cells drain into the superior meatus and if present the supreme meatus.

Anatomic variations predisposing an individual to sinusitis by narrowing one of the osteomeatal channels can be diagnosed on CT. Additionally, CT can define complications of sinusitis such as polyps, bone destruction or thickening, and inflammatory involvement of the orbit or brain (30). CT scans demonstrate the medial roof of the anterior ethmoid and its anatomic variations. This thin bone contains the anterior ethmoidal artery as it passes from the ethmoid to the olfactory fossa and can be fractured during endoscopic ethmoid surgery (31).

The anatomic variations that could impair sinus drainage and lead to recurrent sinusitis should be noted on CT and include concha bullosa, Haller cells, large ethmoid bulla, uncinate deviation, paradoxically curved middle turbinates, uncinate process bulla, and nasal septal deviation (Figs. 3.8–3.10). A laterally deviated tip of the uncinate process can obstruct the distal infundibulum and hiatus semilunaris. A medially deviated tip may obstruct the middle meatus.

Concha bullosa refers to aerated middle turbinates, which can compress the uncinate process and obstruct the middle meatus and infundibulum (32). Haller cells are ethmoid air cells that extend inferiorly to the ethmoid bullae and lateral onto the roof of the maxillary sinus. They are in continuity with the proximal infundibulum and may narrow the ostium of the maxillary sinus. Ethmoid bulla refers to the pneumatized bony bar running above and posterior to the uncinate process. Large bulla may narrow and obstruct the middle meatus. By extending into the hiatus semilunaris, the bulla can contact the uncinate process and block the infundibulum. In the paradoxically curved middle turbinate, the lateral deviation narrows the middle meatus and compresses the infundibulum.

The ethmoid air cells vary in number and are superimposed on conventional radiographs. As with the maxillary sinuses, the ethmoids are present at birth. Involvement of some ethmoid cells easily overlooked on plain radiography can be detected by CT. Nasal secretions, swollen turbinates, multiple septa' walls, underexposed radiographs, and rotation can cause normal ethmoids to appear clouded on plain radiographs. Focal ethmoid clouding more commonly occurs in the anterior cells but can occur posteriorly as well. Unilateral sphenoid clouding, easily diagnosed on CT, may be impossible to detect on lateral plain radiographs.

In a prospective study of 70 infants and children with recurrent acute sinusitis, plain radiographs were com-

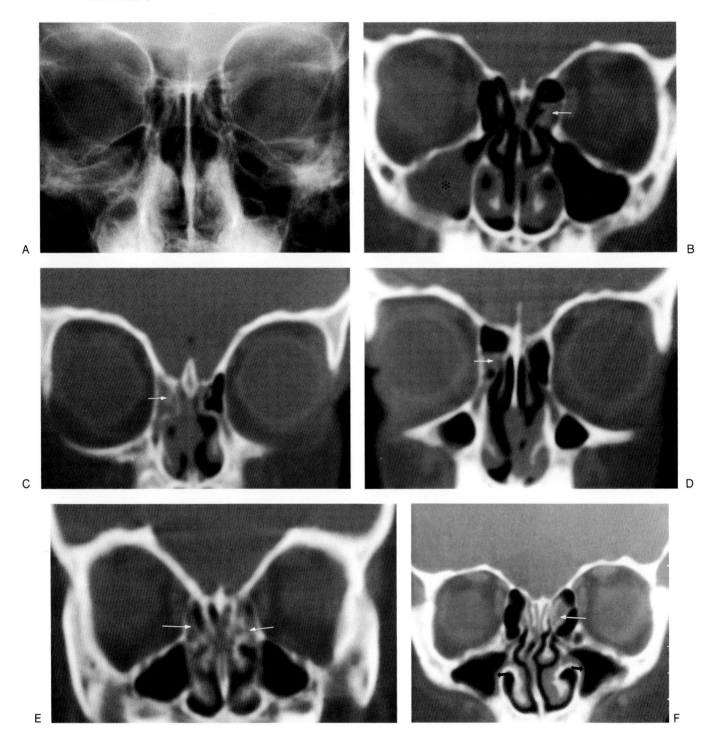

FIG. 3.11. Plain radiographs interpreted as normal but with soft tissue opacification noted on coronal CT examinations in asymptomatic patients on therapy for recurrent sinusitis. **A:** Caldwell projection interpreted as having normal ethmoids. The right maxillary sinus was partially opacified. **B:** A coronal CT in same patient as **(A)**, showing ethmoid bulla clouding on the left (*arrow*) and a retention cyst on the right (*asterisk*). **C–G:** Other examples of abnormal CT scans with ethmoid clouding (*white arrows*) in patients also with normal plain radiographs performed immediately prior to CT scans.

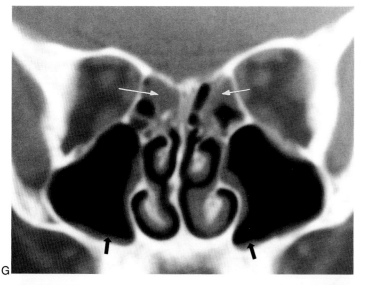

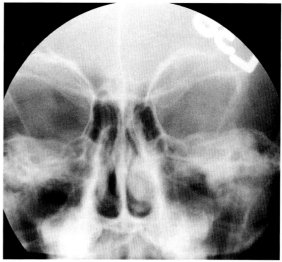

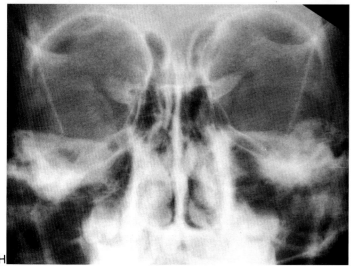

FIG. 3.11. (*Continued*) Parts **(F)** and **(G)** also have maxillary sinus mucous membrane thickening (*black arrows*). **H, I:** Caldwell projections interpreted as normal with focal ethmoid clouding on coronal CT scans (not shown).

pared with coronal CT scans taken within 1 h of one another (19). The CT was considered to be the diagnostic standard. The sinus plain radiographs and coronal CT scans failed to correlate in 74% of the patients. Forty-five percent of patients with normal plain radiographs had abnormalities on CT scan and 34% of those with abnormal plain radiographs had normal CT scans (Figs. 3.11–3.17). In 67% of the patients or in 59% of the evaluated ethmoids, the ethmoids were abnormal on CT scans. Discrepancies in ethmoid disease comparing plain sinus radiographs to CT scans were noted in 25% of patients. When the ethmoids were abnormal the anterior cells were involved 91% of the time. Isolated posterior ethmoid involvement occurred in only 9% of the diseased ethmoids. Maxillary sinuses on coronal sinus CT were abnormal in 64% of the patients. The sphenoid and frontal sinuses on CT scans were abnormal in 31%. Discrepancies in interpreta-

tions of plain radiographs and CT scan were 23% for the maxillary sinus, 26% for the sphenoid sinus, and 16% for the frontal sinus. Discrepancies between plain radiographs and CT scans were more common in the younger age groups. Compared to CT, plain radiographs are unreliable in diagnosing sinus disease in infants and young children as they both overdiagnose and underdiagnose sinus disease. Plain radiographs cannot localize ethmoid disease sufficiently to guide endoscopic sinus surgery (Fig. 3.18). Also, soft tissue clouding in the anterior ethmoids is common in asymptomatic patients with recurrent sinusitis on prolonged therapy (19).

The significance of sinus opacification on CT examinations performed for reasons other than clinical sinus disease is not entirely clear. Diament et al. (33) found that 50% of children undergoing CT examinations had maxillary sinus opacification. Glasier et al.

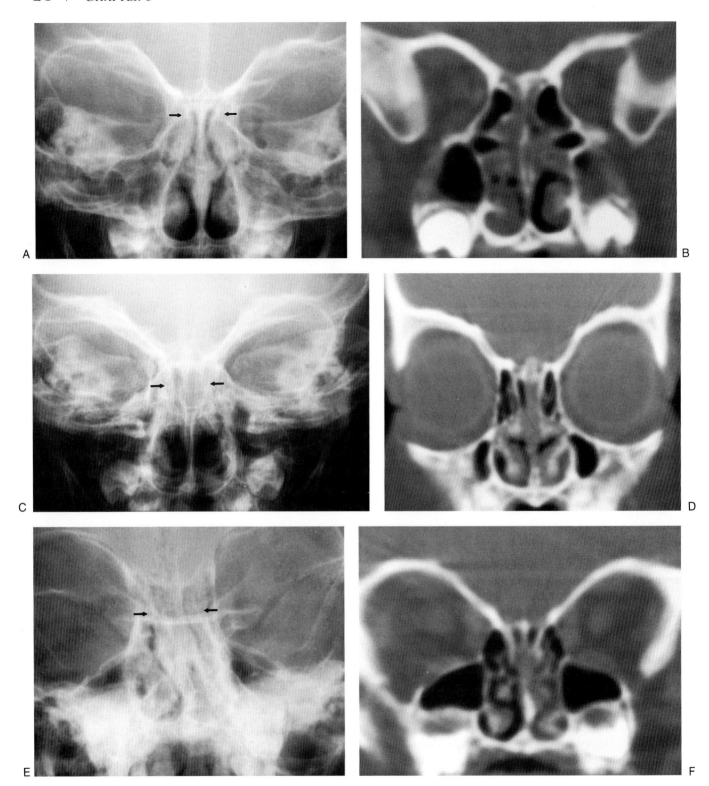

FIG. 3.12. Discrepancies between plain sinus radiographs and coronal CT scans performed within 1 h of one another. Ethmoid sinus clouding (*arrows*) interpreted on plain radiographs (**A**, **C**, and **E**), but with normal corresponding ethmoids on coronal CT examinations (**B**, **D**, and **F**).

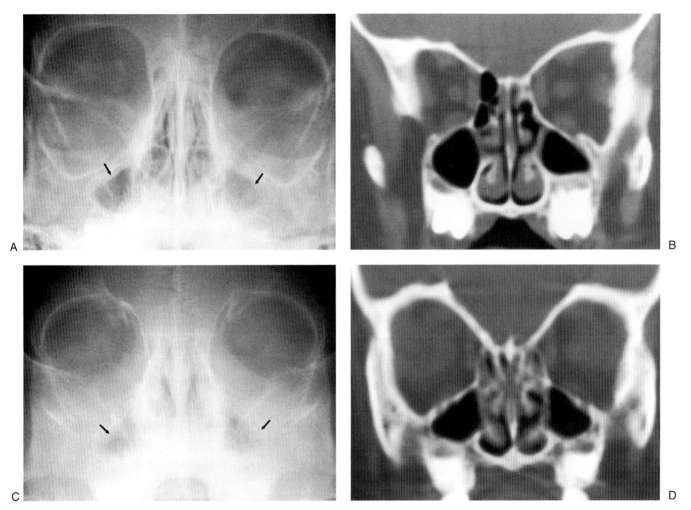

FIG. 3.13. Discrepancies between plain sinus radiographs (**A** and **C**) and coronal CT scans (**B** and **D**) performed within 1 h of one another. Maxillary sinus mucous membrane thickening (*arrows*) interpreted on Waters projections (**A** and **C**) with normal corresponding coronal CT examinations of the maxillary sinuses (**B** and **D**).

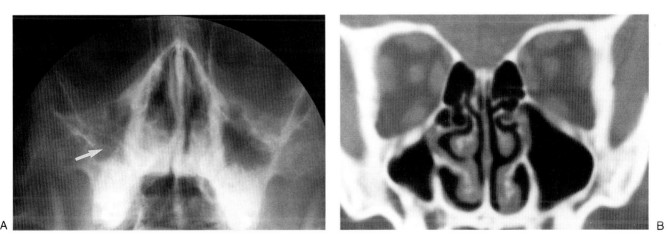

FIG. 3.14. Hypoplasia of the right maxillary sinus simulating disease. **A:** Waters projection showing an apparent clouded right maxillary sinus (*arrow*). **B:** Coronal CT scan performed within 1 h of the plain radiographs shows the small, normally aerated sinus.

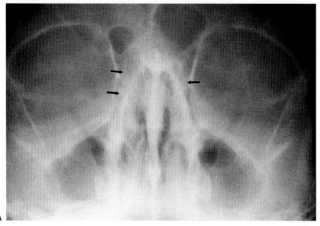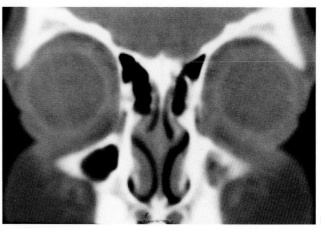

FIG. 3.15. Apparent clouding of anterior ethmoid air cells on Waters projection but with a normal coronal CT scan taken within 1 h of plain radiographs. **A:** Waters projection interpreted as showing anterior ethmoid clouding (*arrows*). **B:** Normal anterior coronal CT scan.

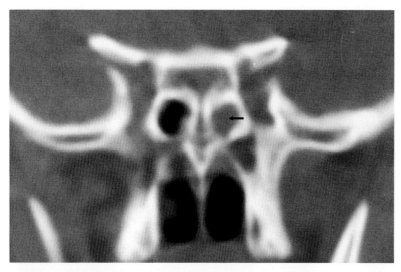

FIG. 3.16. Coronal sinus CT scan demonstrating opacification of the left sphenoid sinus (*arrow*) with minimal soft tissue in the other sphenoid sinus but with normal plain radiographs (not shown).

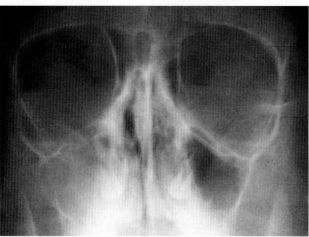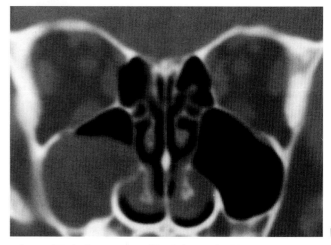

FIG. 3.17. Proven retention cyst in right maxillary sinus simulating an opacified sinus. **A:** Waters projection showing the right maxillary sinus to be opacified. **B:** Coronal sinus CT showing the large retention cyst.

FIG. 3.18. Inability of plain radiographs to localize ethmoid clouding for endoscopic sinus surgery. Waters (**A**) and Caldwell (**B**) projections in a 3-year-old showing partial ethmoidal and complete maxillary sinus opacification. Two scans (**C, D**) of a coronal sinus CT showing focal ethmoid clouding (*arrows*) and maxillary sinus opacification. Right lateral (**E**) and left lateral (**F**) reformatted images demonstrating the areas of ethmoidal involvement (*arrows*). MT, middle turbinate; IT, inferior turbinate; HP, hard palate; A, adenoids; T, tongue.

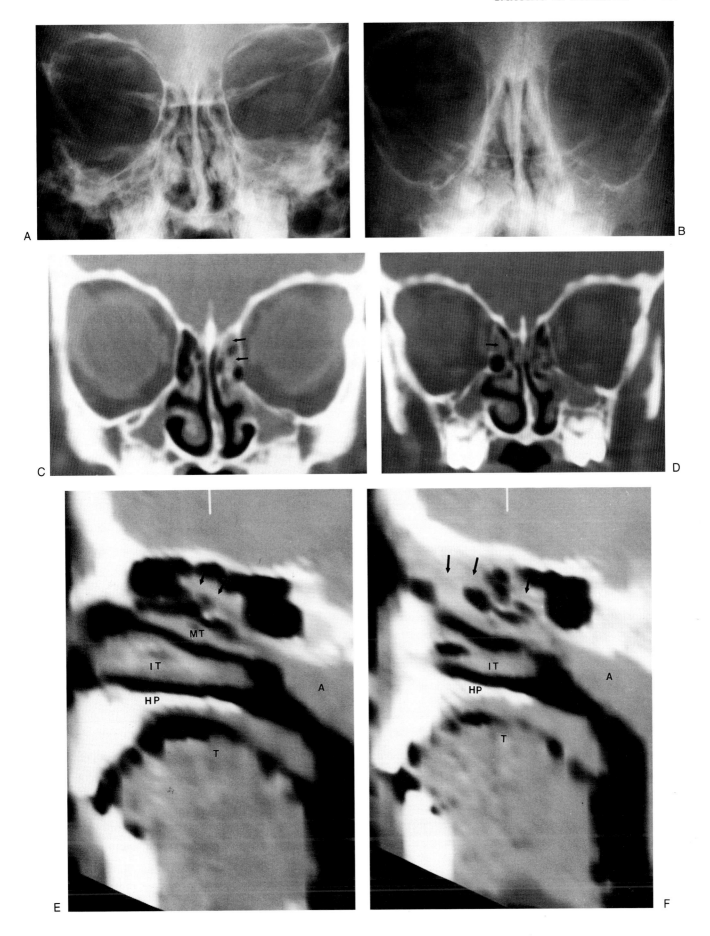

(34) found that 87% of infants less than 1 year of age with a history of a recent upper respiratory infection had opacification of the sinuses. However, 59% of patients without such infections had opacification.

In a prospective CT study of paranasal sinus abnormalities, clouding was found in 18% of asymptomatic patients older than 1 year of age (35). This figure rose to 31% in patients with a recent upper respiratory infection (35). Eleven percent of adults without clinical sinusitis or allergic rhinitis undergoing cranial CT had ethmoid clouding (36).

MAGNETIC RESONANCE

Magnetic resonance imaging (MRI) uses a high-strength magnetic field and a radiofrequency wave to produce cross-sectional images of the paranasal sinuses. Advantages of MRI include its multiplanar display, which enables anatomic formatting in axial (transverse), coronal, and sagittal planes without patient repositioning. CT is usually limited to coronal and axial planes. Dental amalgam does not interfere with MRI image quality.

MRI also has superior soft tissue contrast. Inflammatory disease and free fluid generally have intense signals on T2-weighted images, whereas tumors may have only intermediate signal (37). The increased signal in the mucosa undergoing cyclic volumetric changes in the ethmoids on the T2-weighted images was similar to that seen in inflammatory mucosa (15,38). MRI can also evaluate blood breakdown products in complicating sinonasal hemorrhage and differentiate this hemorrhage from mucosal reaction and sinus effusion (39).

Signal characteristics, however, are not always specific. A low or absent signal on T1-weighted and T2-weighted images can be caused by air, desiccated secretions, mycetomas, acute hemorrhage, calcium, bone, or enamel. When surrounded by material that is hypointense on T1-weighted images and hyperintense on T2-weighted images, differentiation may be impossible (40).

MRI has other serious limitations in the evaluation of acute sinus disease. It is expensive and requires prolonged patient cooperation during lengthy examinations. This latter feature is especially important in the pediatric population. MRI is also contraindicated in patients with aneurysm clips, cardiac pacemakers, and stapedial implants, limitations that should be mentioned but rarely affect children. MRI does not image cortical bone, impairing its ability to evaluate the osteomeatal complex. Marrow signals, however, can be studied. Well demonstrated are the fatty changes that the marrow undergoes prior to pneumatization (41).

Despite its attributes, MRI is best reserved for selected patients in whom refined tissue characterization is essential. CT remains the recommended modality for evaluation of inflammatory disease including fungal infection. The significance of sinus disease when seen on MRI is similar to that of CT. In a study of patients with clinical sinus disease 12 years of age and older, MRI demonstrated the sphenoid sinuses to be abnormal in 6%, the maxillary in 23%, ethmoid in 34%, and the frontals in 16% (42).

In a study involving patients ranging in age from 15 to 85 years, 1 to 2 mm of mucous membrane thickening was seen in 63% of asymptomatic patients (15). In that study, there was no statistical difference between those with clinical symptoms and signs of sinus disease until there was 4 mm or more of mucous membrane thickening. The authors felt that minimal mucosal thickening of the ethmoids may be related to cyclic changes in nasal mucosal volume (15,38). These cyclic changes of increased thickness apparently occur in the ethmoids, but not in the maxillary, frontal, or sphenoid sinuses (38).

Chronically obstructed sinuses usually have secretions that are hypointense on T1-weighted images and hyperintense on T2-weighted images. Variable signal intensities occasionally observed in chronic sinusitis are due to the amount of free water, macromolecular proteins, and the viscosity (43). Some authors have promoted MRI of the paranasal sinuses by offering screening examinations inexpensively (44).

SONOGRAPHY

Somewhat less expensive, sonography of the maxillary sinuses has been recommended by some authors and does have the advantage of using no ionizing radiation (45). The concept of screening sonography is simple in that the fluid-filled maxillary sinus or the membrane thickened sinus will transmit sound and the air-containing sinus will not. However, frequent technical problems in part account for wide discrepancies in reported results. A prospective investigation of 75 patients with a median age of 10 years compared a Waters projection to A-mode sonography (46). The false positive rate of sonography was 39 to 45% depending on criteria for radiographic abnormality; the false negative rate was 42 to 56%. The sensitivity of sonography was 44 to 58% and the specificity was 55 to 61% (46). In another study involving opacified maxillary sinuses shown on radiography, A-mode sonography was abnormal in only 58% (47). In selected patients sonography may be valuable (45). We are skeptical about the application of sonography to sinus disease in children until additional prospective comparative clinical studies are reported. Another major liability of sonography is the lack of ability to image the ethmoid sinuses.

PLURIDIRECTIONAL TOMOGRAPHY

In our practice this technique has been replaced by CT.

ACUTE BACTERIAL SINUSITIS

Acute bacterial sinusitis characteristically produces ill-defined thickening of the mucous membranes, sinus opacification, and air–fluid levels in the involved sinuses on plain films (Figs. 3.19 and 3.20) (48,49). Acute bacterial sinusitis is more difficult to diagnose in infants and children on clinical grounds, but when an upper respiratory infection, purulent nasal secretions, and pain are present, radiographic changes of sinusitis may be found in as many as 75% of patients (50). Bone margins or sinus lamina dura are intact but may be deossified with persistent disease (51). Frank bone destruction favors a more aggressive inflammatory process such as a fungus. Acute bacterial sinusitis is often asymmetric. There may be swelling of the nasal mucosa and turbinates. Wald (52) stated that total opacification, air–fluid levels, and mucous membrane thickening in conjunction with symptoms predicted bacteria in maxillary sinuses in 75% of children over 2 years of age. In acute sinusitis air–fluid levels have greater significance than does mucous membrane thickening. Mucous membrane thickening, especially in younger children, is far less specific for sinusitis than are air–fluid levels. Also, the radiographic diagnosis of sinusitis in older children is more specific. Despite some evidence that fluid can be aspirated from the maxillary sinuses in as many as 39% of children with

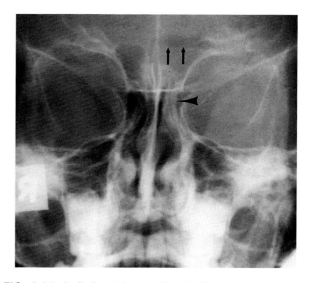

FIG. 3.20. Left frontal sinusitis. A 10-year-old showing opacification of left frontal sinus with an air–fluid level (*arrows*). Some left ethmoid clouding is also noted (*arrowhead*).

normal plain radiographs (18), clear sinuses make acute sinusitis less likely.

The CT evaluation of acute sinusitis may be helpful in evaluating the ethmoid and sphenoid sinuses and the bone. The ethmoid cells may have mucosal thickening or diffuse opacification (Fig. 3.21). With the administration of intravenous contrast the mucosa enhances, sparing the central mucoid secretions (Fig. 3.22). On CT, mucosal thickening may occasionally be polypoid (53–55).

On CT, air–fluid levels are best seen on direct coronal projections with the patient prone or supine (Fig. 3.23). Air–fluid levels may also occur from antral lavage and persist for 3 or 4 days, or from sinus hemorrhage as a result of trauma, hemophilia, or other co-

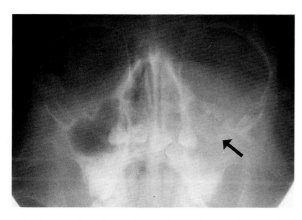

FIG. 3.19. Acute left maxillary sinusitis. The left maxillary sinus is opacified (*arrow*).

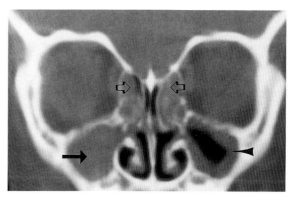

FIG. 3.21. Acute sinusitis. Coronal CT scan demonstrates an opacified right maxillary sinus (*arrow*), mucosal thickening in the left maxillary sinus (*arrowhead*), and bilateral ethmoid opacification (*open arrows*).

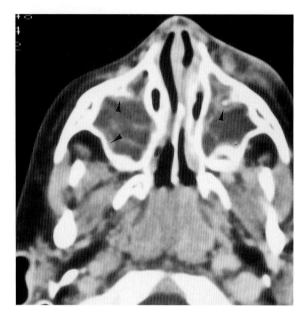

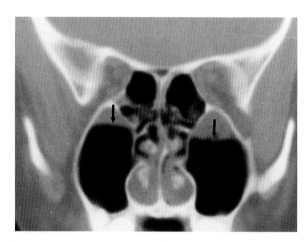

FIG. 3.23. Acute sinusitis. Coronal CT scan with bilateral maxillary air–fluid levels (*arrows*). Examination done with head down.

FIG. 3.22. Acute sinusitis. Axial CT scan shows contrast enhancement of the mucosal membranes (*arrowheads*) and low-density contents in bilateral opacified maxillary sinuses.

agulation disorders. Differentiating clinically acute infections from chronic changes may be difficult. Clinically, sinusitis should resolve in a few weeks and radiographic documentation of clearing is recommended. CT scans can distinguish conditions such as thalassemia (Fig. 3.24) and hypoplastic sinuses (Fig. 3.14), which simulate sinusitis on plain radiographs.

The most characteristic MRI appearance of the edematous mucosa and fluid is hypointensity on T1-weighted images and hyperintensity on T2-weighted images (Fig. 3.25). The role of the intravenous contrast agent gadopentetate dimeglumine is unclear but may help in evaluating disease outside the sinuses.

Complications of acute sinusitis such as orbital abscess, meningitis, cerebral abscess, epidural and subdural empyema, cavernous sinus thrombosis, and osteomyelitis are discussed separately.

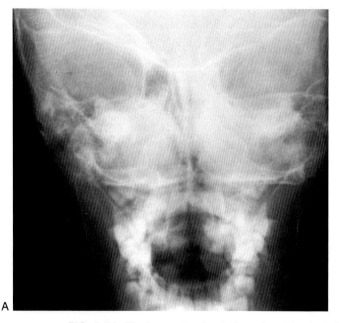

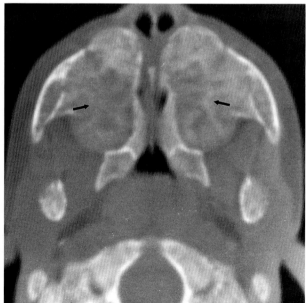

FIG. 3.24. Thalassemia simulating sinusitis. **A:** Caldwell projection demonstrates maxillary sinus and left ethmoid opacification. **B:** Axial CT scan shows maxillary sinuses (*arrows*) replaced by bone marrow.

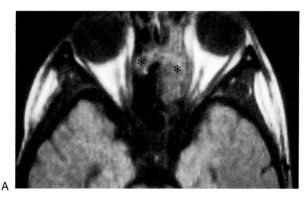
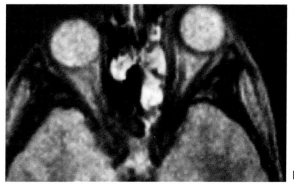

FIG. 3.25. Acute sinusitis. **A:** T1-weighted MR image with medium signal intensity material in the left ethmoid and focally in the right ethmoid sinuses (*asterisks*). **B:** T2-weighted MR image. The ethmoid sinusitis has an increased signal intensity.

RECURRENT ACUTE SINUSITIS

Recurrent acute sinusitis, especially in younger children, is a common problem in pediatrics. The osteomeatal complex is the key to this recurrent disease. Persistent or residual changes in the sinuses, especially the ethmoids, are seen on CT scans in over two-thirds of patients with recurrent sinusitis despite the absence of clinical signs or symptoms of disease (Fig. 3.26) (19).

ALLERGIC RHINITIS/SINUSITIS

Allergic rhinitis is mediated by IgE with swelling of the nasal mucosal membranes. The mucosa of the sinuses is also involved. Production of seromucous secretions increases. The membrane edema can block sinus drainage, resulting in a complicating bacterial sinusitis (56). Sinusitis associated with allergy tends to be diffuse and symmetric with polyp formation. Nasal

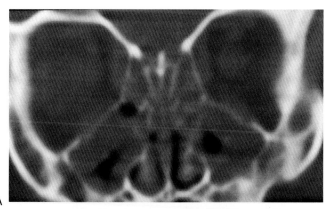
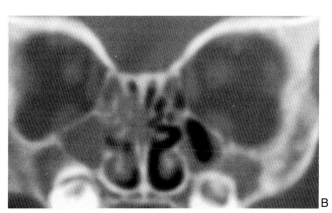
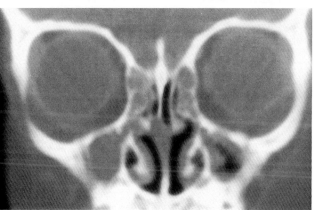

FIG. 3.26. Residual sinus opacification as shown in three patients after months of therapy including antibiotics. Coronal CT scans (**A–C**). Ethmoid and maxillary soft tissue disease can be seen.

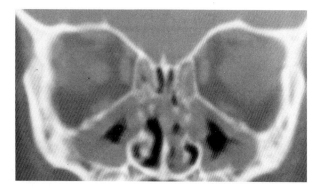

FIG. 3.27. Allergic sinusitis. Coronal CT scan demonstrates polypoid mucosal thickening in the nasal cavity and maxillary sinuses. The ethmoid sinuses are opacified.

polyps are not uncommon. Polyps may develop in the maxillary sinus adjacent to the ostium and later spread into the nose. That allergic mucosal swelling unassociated with obstruction or superimposed infection produces symptomatic sinus disease has not been estab-

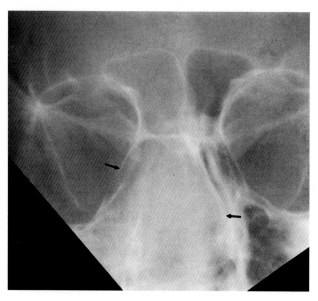

FIG. 3.28. Allergic polyposis. There is expansion of the right nasal cavity and right ethmoids (*arrows*). The right frontal sinus is opacified along with the right ethmoid.

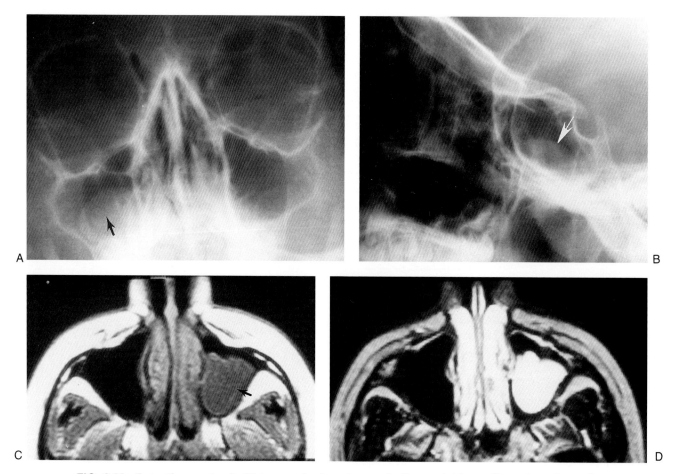

FIG. 3.29. Retention cysts. **A:** Waters projection demonstrating a right maxillary sinus (*arrow*). **B:** Lateral radiograph demonstrates a mass (*arrow*) in the sphenoid sinus. **C:** T1-weighted MR image shows a low signal in the left maxillary mass (*arrow*). **D:** The T2-weighted MR image shows a high signal.

lished. Prolonged disease can result in expansion of the paranasal sinuses with a secondary hypertelorism, malar fullness, and brow prominence. Children with sinonasal allergies have a high incidence of sinus opacification and in one study of 70 such children over 50% had abnormal sinus radiographs (16).

Plain radiographs demonstrate partial or complete opacification of all sinuses (54). Bacterial sinusitis is more frequently asymmetric (57). Contrast enhanced CT demonstrates opacified sinuses with enhancing mucosal thickening that may be irregular (Fig. 3.27). Nasal polyps, less common in bacterial sinusitis, are helpful features of allergic sinusitis. Nasal polyps are also common in patients with cystic fibrosis. Air–fluid levels are less common in allergic sinus disease. Despite published statements concerning the radiographic differential diagnostic features of allergic and bacterial sinusitis, no definitive data exist and the sensitivity and specificity of the differential radiographic diagnosis are unknown. Marked allergic polyposis can produce an enlarged sinus. This appearance has been termed polypoid mucocele (Fig. 3.28).

MUCUS RETENTION CYSTS

Mucus retention cysts, which are noninflammatory lesions, must be differentiated from inflammatory polyps (53,58). The retention cyst is probably a distended mucus gland. Synonyms include a nonsecreting cyst, noninflammatory cyst, serous cyst, or mucus gland cyst. Although seen in approximately 10% of the population, children are affected less frequently. They are most common in the inferior recesses of the maxillary sinus but also can occur in the frontal and sphenoid sinuses (Figs. 3.29A,B). Plain radiographs are almost always sufficient for a diagnosis, assuming that the remainder of the sinus is normal. When there is appreciable mucous membrane thickening, a retention cyst cannot be differentiated from polypoid mucosal thickening on plain radiographs.

CT is helpful in evaluating large lesions that otherwise may not be seen fully on plain radiographs. A cap of air positioned superiorly over the convexity of a rounded, low-density, homogeneous soft tissue lesion suggests a retention cyst rather than a mucocele or free fluid (Fig. 3.17). On MRI, mucus retention cysts are usually hypointense on T1-weighted images and hyperintense on T2-weighted images (Figs. 3.29C,D).

MUCOCELE AND PYOMUCOCELES

A mucocele is a smoothly marginated enlargement of a sinus due to an obstructed ostium of a paranasal sinus. Radiographic evidence of bone destruction or marked soft tissue swelling should suggest pyomuco-

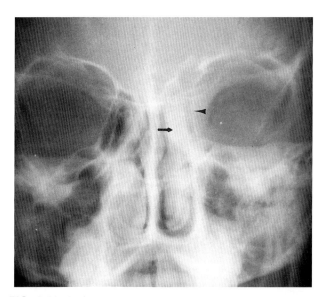

FIG. 3.30. Left ethmoid pyomucocele. There is opacification of the left ethmoid (*arrow*) and adjacent frontal sinus with poor definition of the left medial orbital wall (*arrowhead*).

cele (Figs. 3.30 and 3.31). When sinus expansion and bone destruction are not apparent, the findings may simulate sinusitis. Mucoceles contain mucoid material and desquamated epithelium with variable CT densities. Sixty-five percent of these lesions occur in the frontal sinuses. The second most frequent site is the ethmoids (25%), followed by the sphenoid and max-

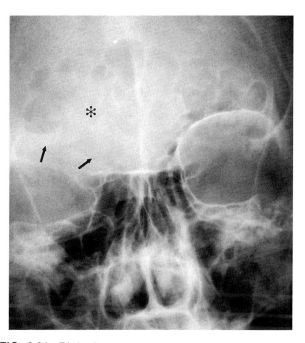

FIG. 3.31. Right frontal pyomucocele. The right frontal sinus (*asterisk*) is opacified. The right orbital roof is eroded and depressed (*arrows*). The left frontal sinus is also partially opacified.

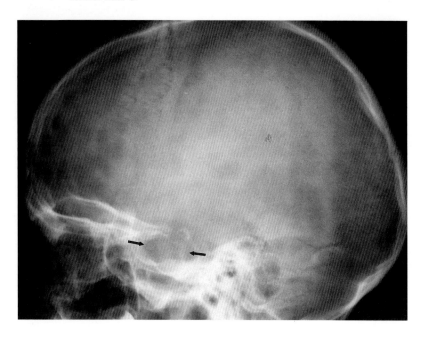

FIG. 3.32. Sphenoid mucocele. Lateral radiograph shows extensive bony erosion of sphenoid (*arrows*) including the sella.

illary sinuses (10%) (59). Although rare, sphenoid mucoceles are silent until they involve adjacent vital organs and structures. They may become quite large (Figs. 3.32 and 3.33) and may extend into the ethmoid sinuses or brain. The adjacent carotid arteries also can be displaced. Lesions of the frontal sinus may extend infralaterally into the orbit or posteriorly into the cerebrum.

The predominant radiographic finding is that of increased density of the sinus with expansion of the walls of the sinuses. The mucoperiosteum will be demineralized. Frank bone destruction can also occur (Fig. 3.32). CT remains the preferred modality for diagnosis. CT superbly demonstrates bony expansion (Fig. 3.34). The fluid within the sinus is low density and the mucosa is often hypertrophied. Polyps may be the cause of the obstruction that prompted mucocele formation. However, expansion of a sinus by polyps can cause similar plain radiographic findings as a mucocele. Since mucoceles do not enhance, a thin rim of enhancement suggests a complicating pyomucocele (Fig. 3.34) (60).

Two MRI patterns are seen with mucoceles. The first is a decreased signal on the T1- and T2-weighted sequences. Inflamed mucosa around the periphery of the sinuses is hypointense on the T1-weighted sequence and hyperintense on the T2-weighted se-

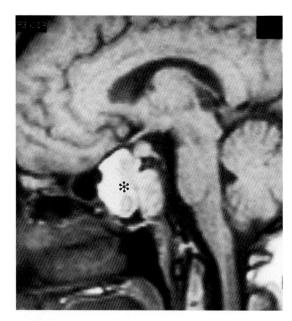

FIG. 3.33. Sphenoid mucocele. Proton density-weighted MR image shows an increased signal intensity mass in the sphenoid (*asterisk*).

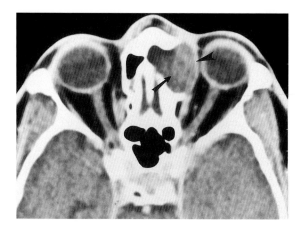

FIG. 3.34. Ethmoid pyomucocele. Axial CT scan shows erosion of the left ethmoid by an expansile soft tissue mass (*arrow*) and some rim enhancement (*arrowhead*) after contrast administration.

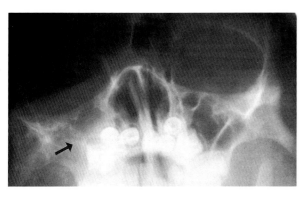

FIG. 3.35. Actinomycosis. Waters projection shows an opacified right maxillary sinus in a Vietnamese boy (*arrow*).

quences. This pattern is most frequently seen with hard dehydrated material within the sinus (58). A second pattern is that of increased signal on the T2-weighted sequence and some increase on the T1-weighted and proton density-weighted sequences (Fig. 3.33). This pattern corresponds to lesions that are isointense or hypointense on CT.

AGGRESSIVE FUNGAL SINUSITIS

Mucormycosis, actinomycosis, and aspergillosis frequently produce an aggressive sinusitis in debilitated, immunosuppressed, or ketoacidotic patients. Mucormycosis usually originates in the nasal cavity or paranasal sinus and can extend into the deep cranial facial

structures of the orbit, cavernous sinuses, and brain (61,62). These organisms invade blood vessels and produce a purulent arteritis with intracranial dissemination.

Plain sinus radiographs demonstrate sinus opacification, occasional bony wall destruction, and evidence of extension beyond the paranasal sinuses (Fig. 3.35) (63). Air–fluid levels are uncommon (64). The mucosal thickening may be nodular. Involvement of the frontal and sphenoid sinus is uncommon.

CT demonstrates extension into deep tissues with loss of the normal fat planes in the orbit, infratemporal fossa, and pterygopalatine fossa (Fig. 3.36) (64). High-intensity material may be seen in the sinuses (Fig. 3.37A). Increased CT density of the orbital apical fat or orbital apex signals disease that may be typical on CT for fungal sinusitis. With orbital involvement, the medial rectus is widened and displaced laterally. The optic nerve may be enlarged and displaced laterally with an indistinct margin as it enters the apex (61). Infarction, cerebritis, and abscess may develop when intracranial vessels are involved.

Angiography may be helpful on occasion because of the tendency of mucormyocosis to proliferate in the muscle walls of vessels, producing an arteritis with thrombosis and infarction (65). Angiography may show narrowing or occlusion of the cavernous carotid artery or occlusion of the ophthalmic artery. Cavernous sinus thrombosis is less common than thrombosis of the cavernous portion of the internal carotid artery (62).

Unlike acute bacterial sinusitis involving the orbit, subperiosteal abscesses are uncommon in fungal sinusitis (54). From the maxilla the disease extends into

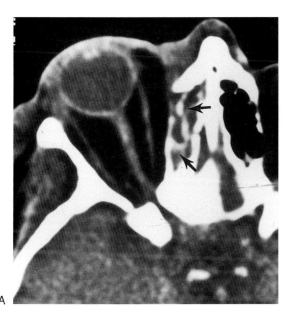

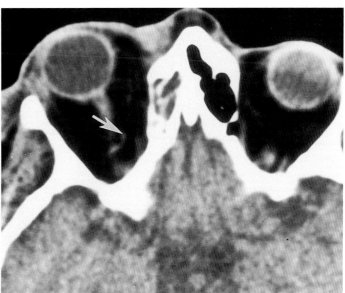

A B

FIG. 3.36. Mucormycosis in a patient with leukemia. Axial CT scans. **A:** Right ethmoid opacification (*arrows*) and soft tissue swelling in the right periorbital tissues are shown. **B:** There is soft tissue extension (*arrow*) to the orbital cone.

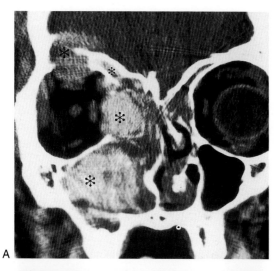

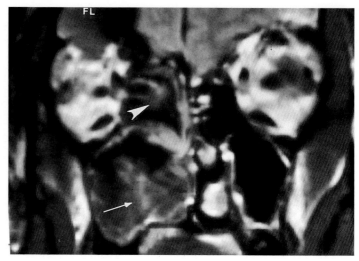

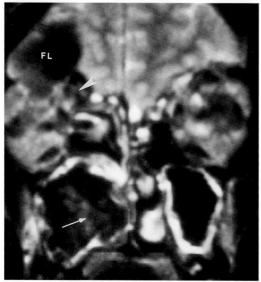

FIG. 3.37. Aggressive aspergillosis. **A:** Coronal CT scan shows a high attenuation material in the right maxillary, right ethmoid, and right frontal sinuses and the right frontal lobe (*asterisks*). **B:** T1-weighted MR image demonstrates a moderate signal intensity in the right maxillary antrum (*arrow*) along with low signal material in the right ethmoid (*arrowhead*) and right frontal lobe (FL). **C:** T2-weighted MR image shows low signal intensity within right maxillary (*arrow*), ethmoid, and frontal (*arrowhead*) sinuses and right frontal lobe (FL).

the infratemporal fossa and through the superior orbital fissure into the middle cranial fossa.

On T2-weighted MRI sequences, fungal sinusitis can be isointense to hypointense compared to normal mucosa (Fig. 3.37). This decreased signal may be due to iron and manganese within the fungus (66).

EXTRAMUCOSAL OR ALLERGIC ASPERGILLUS SINUSITIS

Extramucosal or allergic aspergillus sinusitis tends to occur in patients who have nasal polyps. Progressive expansion of the sinus disease leads to facial deformity (67). Asthma or other allergies may be present. By plain radiographs the sinuses are typically expanded and opacified (67). On CT dense concretions within the sinus containing hydroxyapatite and calcium sulfate within areas of necrosis of the mycetoma are usually seen (68). Areas of signal void may be seen on the

T2-weighted sequence of the MRI. At surgery the sinuses are packed with greenish-black inspissated mucin-containing Charcot–Leyden crystals, aggregates of degenerated eosinophils, and patchy calcification. This suggests an allergic reaction similar to allergic bronchopulmonary aspergillosis. Three other forms of aspergillosis of the sinus include the fulminant variety with soft tissue invasion in immune compromised hosts; an indolent, slowly progressive, but still invasive form; and a localized noninvasive form similar to a pulmonary mycetoma.

CHRONIC SINUSITIS

Chronic sinusitis is defined as sinusitis with symptoms and findings persisting for greater than 3 weeks despite treatment (16,48,52). However, radiographic changes associated with chronic sinusitis are due to much more long-standing disease. Chronic sinusitis causes an osteoblastic response in the affected sinus walls. Most frequently, the maxillary sinuses are involved. The sinus is usually decreased in size although resultant polyps may actually increase antral size (69). Foci of irregular bone thinning, particularly on the nasal surface of the maxillary sinus, may be seen.

GRANULOMATOUS SINUSITIS

Sarcoidosis, Wegener's granulomatosis, and midline granuloma can produce similar changes as chronic sinusitis but with more extensive bone destruction. These processes usually begin in the nasal septum (54).

Plain radiographs show opacified sinuses and expanded or destroyed bony margins. The more bone destruction evident, the more likely the disease is midline granuloma rather than Wegener's or sarcoid. The disease is usually bilateral and symmetrically located about the nasal septum. Extension into the maxillary, ethmoid, and sphenoid sinuses is often present. Frontal sinus involvement is uncommon. The findings on CT and MRI are similar and nonspecific for these entities. Biopsy is often necessary for precise diagnosis.

CONDITIONS ASSOCIATED WITH PARANASAL SINUSITIS

Cystic Fibrosis

Chronic sinusitis is common in cystic fibrosis (70–72). The frequency of chronic sinusitis in cystic fibrosis varies from 93 to 100% in several series (72). The sinus may be opacified without any clinical signs or symptoms of sinus disease (Fig. 3.38). Bilateral nasal polyps are very uncommon in small children without cystic fibrosis. Their presence should suggest the diagnosis of cystic fibrosis (71). Polypoid mucoceles similar to those found in allergic sinusitis may occur.

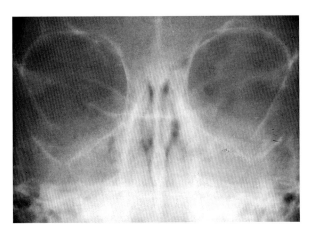

FIG. 3.38. Cystic fibrosis. A Waters projection shows opacified maxillary sinuses in a 3-year-old. There were no sinus directed signs or symptoms.

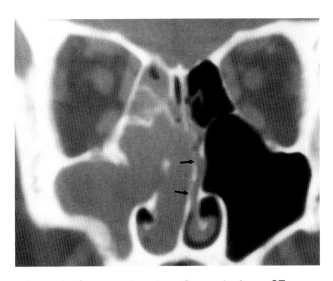

FIG. 3.39. Nasoantral polyp. Coronal sinus CT scan shows opacification of the right maxillary sinus and extension of mass into the nasal cavity and bowing of the nasal septum (*arrows*).

Immune Deficiency Syndromes

Examples of some of the conditions associated with congenital immune deficiencies include ataxia-telangiectasia and immotile-cilia syndrome. They are characteristically associated with sinus opacification. In addition, patients with immunosuppressive disorders, including acquired immunodeficiency syndrome, can develop paranasal sinus disease. When fungal infections occur, the radiographic finding of bone destruction may suggest an aggressive process.

Choanal Polyps

Choanal or antrochoanal polyps are lesions characteristically seen in young males. They are not associated with generalized polyps or allergy. They begin in the maxillary antrum and extend into the nose posteriorly to the posterior choana. The maxillary or ethmoid sinuses can be expanded (Fig. 3.39). On CT, these polyps do not enhance significantly and do not extend into the pterygopalatine fossa beyond the nasopharynx.

COMPLICATIONS OF SINUSITIS

Orbital Cellulitis and Abscess

An orbital abscess or cellulitis occurs most frequently from ethmoid sinusitis and less frequently from maxillary sinusitis or frontal sinusitis and is more common than intracranial extensions (10,73,74). Contributing factors to orbital spread of paranasal sinus

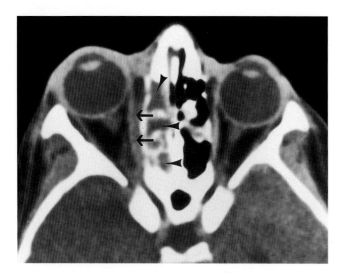

FIG. 3.40. Orbital cellulitis. Axial CT scan. There is an opacified right ethmoid sinus (*arrowheads*) with edema of medial extraconal fat (*arrows*) and lateral displacement of the medial rectus muscle.

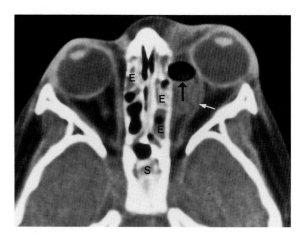

FIG. 3.42. Orbital cellulitis. Axial CT scan. The ethmoid (E) and sphenoid (S) sinuses are opacified. An air–fluid level (*arrow*) indicates a frank left subperiosteal abscess. The left medial rectus muscle (*white arrow*) is displaced laterally.

infection include communication between these anatomic regions via valveless veins and the thinness of the lamina papyracea separating the ethmoids from the orbit. Findings detected by CT are orbital edema (Fig. 3.40), cellulitis including muscle thickening (Figs. 3.41 and 3.45A), or abscess (Fig. 3.42). Inflammatory disease extending from the ethmoid can be subperiosteal, extraconal (Fig. 3.43), or intraconal. Plain radiographs show the sinus opacification although the bone destruction and extrasinus extension are not well shown. Contrast enhanced CT is excellent and can separate preseptal from postseptal inflammatory disease.

Subperiosteal inflammation may slightly enhance following intravenous administration of contrast. A

subperiosteal process is hemispherically shaped and abuts the periosteum. Only the inflammatory margins of a subperiosteal abscess will enhance. The adjacent medial rectus muscle is often edematous and enlarged. Abscesses may occur either in the extraconal or intraconal spaces as well. The intraconal inflammatory disease obliterates the crisp outline of the optic nerve and increases the density of the surrounding intraconal fat. Infection also can extend into the cavernous sinus.

Osteomyelitis

Although maxillary osteomyelitis has been reported as a complication of acute maxillary sinusitis, it is not

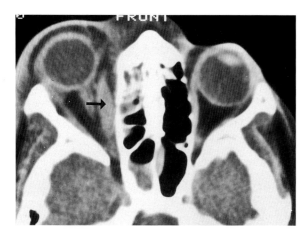

FIG. 3.41. Orbital cellulitis. Axial CT. The right ethmoid and sphenoid sinuses are opacified and there is marked thickening of right medial rectus muscle (*arrow*).

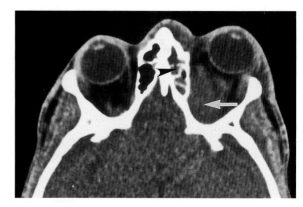

FIG. 3.43. Orbital cellulitis. A proven extraconal abscess (*arrow*) in the left orbit. Left ethmoid opacification from sinusitis is present (*arrowhead*).

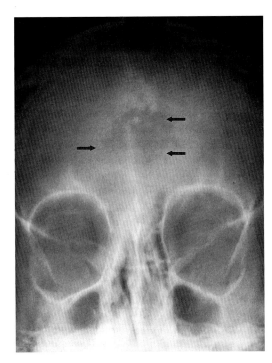

FIG. 3.44. Frontal sinusitis. An 8-year-old with opacified frontal sinuses and an area of destruction (*arrows*) in the bone above the frontal sinuses. The anterior ethmoids were also involved.

cation of the sinus walls or destruction slightly removed from the involved sinus (Fig. 3.44).

Subdural and Epidural Empyema

The most frequent sinus associated with subdural empyema is the infected frontal sinus (75). The absence of dural perforation and frontal osteomyelitis in some cases suggests that communicating veins are the routes of spread. Subdural and epidural empyemas may be difficult to differentiate. Perifalcine collections are subdural in location. Epidural collections tend to remain localized and strip away the dura (Fig. 3.45). Subdural collections tend to be more widespread (77). Extracerebral fluid collections compress the adjacent sulci. Infection can also spread through an eroded posterior wall of the sinus into the epidural space (77). There are no reliable CT or MRI signs that distinguish purulent from nonpurulent collections (78). Vasogenic brain edema is usually not present adjacent to these collections. Therefore adjacent brain displaying decreased density on CT or increased signal on T2-weighted sequences on MRI suggests either cerebritis or ischemia.

common. Osteomyelitis complicates frontal sinusitis more commonly. However, this is rarer than associated epidural or subdural empyema (75,76). The infection spreads to the adjacent narrow spaces of the frontal bone. The frontal swelling can be called Pott's puffy tumor and was described in the 1700s. The plain radiographs show the involved sinus to be opacified. Bone destruction is best shown on CT although plain radiographs may show frank destruction or deossifi-

Meningitis

Meningitis is an uncommon complication of sinus inflammatory disease unless it occurs secondary to extracerebral inflammatory disease. Meningitis is most often seen following ethmoid or sphenoid sinusitis. A contrast enhanced CT examination may show meningeal enhancement. MRI is more sensitive for such meningeal disease (78).

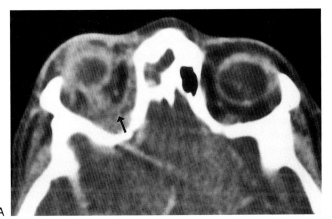

A

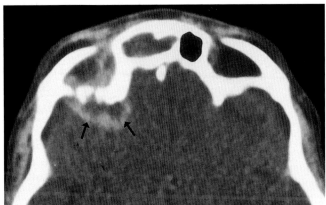

B

FIG. 3.45. Epidural abscess. **A:** Axial CT scan. Sinusitis involving right ethmoid and frontal sinuses with orbital cellulitis (*arrow*). **B:** Axial CT scan. Contrast enhancing dura outlines a discrete epidural collection adjacent to right orbitofrontal plate (*arrows*).

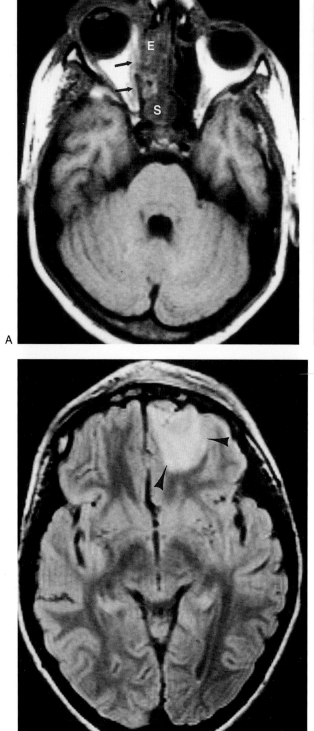

FIG. 3.46. Frontal cerebritis and orbital cellulitis. **A:** T1-weighted MR image shows moderate signal intensity in right ethmoid (E) and sphenoid (S) from sinusitis. There is adjacent orbital cellulitis (*arrows*). **B:** T2-weighted MR image with increased signal intensity from inflammation in the right ethmoid and sphenoid sinus and right orbit (*arrows*). **C:** Proton density-weighted MR image with contralateral frontal cerebritis (*arrowheads*).

Brain Abscess

Frontal sinusitis is the leading cause of frontal lobe abscess or cerebritis (Fig. 3.46) (78). The posterior wall of the frontal sinus is only half the thickness of the anterior wall (79). Brain abscesses from sinusitis are low density on CT with enhancing rims that are usually less than 5 mm in thickness (78). On MRI the wall is isointense on T1-weighted sequences and markedly hypointense on T2-weighted sequences (Fig. 3.37C). The center is hypointense on the T1-weighted sequence and hyperintense on the T2-weighted sequence. Marked ring enhancement follows the intravenous injection of gadopentetate dimeglumine.

Other complications include cavernous sinus thrombosis and the superior orbital fissure syndrome. Infection usually spreads to the cavernous sinus through the orbital veins from orbital cellulitis or from the adjacent sphenoid sinus.

REFERENCES

1. Kuhn JP. Editorial. Imaging of the paranasal sinuses: current status. *J Allergy Clin Immunol* 1986;77:6–8.
2. Waters CA, Waldron CW. Roentgenology of the accessory nasal sinuses describing a modification of the occipito-frontal position. *AJR* 1915;2:633–639.
3. Caldwell EW. Skiagraphy of the accessory sinuses of the nose. *AJR* 1918;5:569–574.
4. Axelsson A, Jensen C. The roentgenologic demonstration of sinusitis. *AJR* 1974;122:621–627.
5. Ilkka K, Matti R. Occipito-meatal side projection radiography in childhood maxillary sinusitis. *Int J Pediatr Otorhinolaryngol* 1990;18:221–225.
6. Kuijpers D, Blickman JG, Camps JA. The five degree rule: optimization of the paranasal sinus examination of children. *Radiology* 1984;152:814.
7. Dolan KD. Paranasal sinus radiology, part 2A: ethmoidal sinuses. *Head Neck Surg* 1982;4:486–498.
8. Maresh MM, Washburn AH. Paranasal sinuses from birth to late adolescence: size of paranasal sinuses as observed on routine posteroanterior roentgenograms. *Am J Dis Child* 1940;60:841–861.
9. Odita JC, Akamaguna AI, Ogisi FO, Amu OD, Ugbodaga CI. Pneumatisation of the maxillary sinus in normal and symptomatic children. *Pediatr Radiol* 1986;16:365–367.
10. Towbin R, Han BK, Kaufman RA, Burke M. Post-septal cellulitis; CT in diagnosis and management. *Radiology* 1986;158:735–737.
11. Dolan KD. Paranasal sinus radiology, part 3A: sphenoid sinus. *Head Neck Surg* 1982;5:164–176.
12. Shopfner CE, Rossi JO. Roentgen evaluation of the paranasal sinuses in children. *AJR* 1973;118:176–186.
13. Uhari M, Lamring P, Kouvalainen K, Akerblom H. Incidence of radiological abnormalities in the maxillary sinuses of children. *Duodecim* 1977;93:327–329.
14. Kovatch AL, Wald ER, Ledesma-Medina J, Chiponis DM, Bedingfield B. Maxillary sinus radiographs in children with nonrespiratory complaints. *Pediatrics* 1984;73:306–308.
15. Rak KM, Newell John D, Yakes WF, Damiano MA, Luethke JM. Paranasal sinuses on MR images of the brain: significance of mucosal thickening. *AJR* 1991;156:381–384.
16. Rachelefsky GS, Katz RM, Siegel SC. Chronic sinusitis in the allergic child. *Pediatr Clin North Am* 1988;35:1091–1101.
17. Adinoff AD, Cummings NP. Sinusitis and its relationship to asthma. *Pediatr Ann* 1989;18:785–790.
18. Watt-Boolsen S, Karle A. The clinical use of radiological examination of the maxillary sinuses. *Clin Otolaryngol* 1977;2:41–43.
19. McAlister WH, Lusk R, Muntz HR. Comparison of plain radiographs and coronal CT scan in infants and children with recurrent sinusitis. *AJR* 1989;153:1259–1264.
20. Lusk RP, Lazar RH, Muntz HR. The diagnosis and treatment of recurrent and chronic sinusitis in children. *Pediatr Clin North Am* 1989;36:1411–1421.
21. Kloppers SP. Endoscopic examination of the nose and results of functional endoscopic sinus surgery in 50 patients. *SAMT* 1987;72:622–624.
22. Zinreich SJ, Kennedy DW, Gayler BW. Computed tomography of nasal cavity and paranasal sinuses: an evaluation of anatomy for endoscopic sinus surgery. *Clear Images* 1988;January:2–10.
23. Zinreich SJ, Kennedy DW, Rosenbaum AE, Gayler BW, Kumar AJ, Stammberger H. Paranasal sinuses: CT imaging requirements for endoscopic surgery. *Radiology* 1987;163:769–775.
24. Pollei S, Harnsberger HR. The radiologic evaluation of the sinonasal region. *Postgrad Radiol* 1989;9:242–266.
25. Som PM, Lawson W, Biller HF, Lanzieri CF. Ethmoid sinus disease: CT evaluation in 400 cases. Part I. Nonsurgical patients. *Radiology* 1986;159:591–597.
26. Jorgensen RA. The use of diagrams in the documentation of endoscopic and CT scan findings in ostiomeatal sinus disease. VIII ISAN International Symposium at Johns Hopkins University School of Medicine, 1989.
27. Terrier F, Weber W, Ruefenacht D, Porcellini B. Anatomy of the ethmoid: CT endoscopic and macroscopic. *AJNR* 1985;6:77–84.
28. Thawley SE. Endoscopic sinus surgery. A functional approach. *Mo Med* 1987;84:237–241.
29. Wallace R, Salagar JE, Cowles S. The relationship between frontal sinus drainage and osteomeatal complex disease: a CT study in 217 patients. *AJNR* 1990;11:183–186.
30. Bilaniuk LT, Zimmerman RA. Computed tomography in evaluation of the paranasal sinuses. *Radiol Clin North Am* 1982;20:51–66.
31. Kainz J, Stammberger H. The roof of the anterior ethmoid: a place of least resistance in the skull base. *Am J Rhinol* 1989;3:191–199.
32. Zinreich SJ, Mattox DE, Kennedy DW, Chisholm HL, Diffley DM, Rosenbaum AE. Concha bullosa: CT evaluation. *J Comput Assist Tomogr* 1988;12:778–784.
33. Diament MJ, Senac MO, Gilsanz V, Baker S, Gillespie T, Larsson S. Prevalence of incidental paranasal sinuses opacification in pediatric patients: a CT study. *J Comput Assist Tomogr* 1987;11:426–431.
34. Glasier CM, Mallory GB, Steele RW. Significance of opacification of maxillary and ethmoid sinuses in infants. *J Pediatr* 1989;114:45–50.
35. Glasier CM, Ascher DP, Williams KD. Incidental paranasal sinus abnormalities on CT of children: clinical correlation. *AJNR* 1986;7:861–864.
36. Duvoisin B, Agrifoglio A. Prevalence of ethmoid sinus abnormalities on brain CT of asymptomatic adults. *AJNR* 1989;10:599–601.
37. Som PM, Shapiro MD, Biller HF, Sasaki C, Lawson W. Sinonasal tumors and inflammatory tissues: differentiation with MR imaging. *Radiology* 1988;167:803–808.
38. Zinreich SJ, Kennedy DW, Kumar AJ, Rosenbaum AE, Arrington JA, Johns ME. MR imaging of normal nasal cycle: comparison with sinus pathology. *J Comput Assist Tomogr* 1988;12:1014–1019.
39. Zimmerman RA, Bilaniuk LT, Hackney DB, Goldberg HI, Grossman RI. Paranasal sinus hemorrhage: evaluation with MR imaging. *Radiology* 1987;162:499–503.
40. Som PM, Dillon WP, Curtin HD, Fullerton GD, Lidov M. Hypointense paranasal sinus foci: differential diagnosis with MR imaging and relation to CT findings. *Radiology* 1990;176:777–781.
41. Aoki S, Dillon WP, Barkovich AJ, Norman D. Marrow conversion before pneumatization of the sphenoid sinus: assessment with MR imaging. *Radiology* 1989;172:373–375.
42. Digre KB, Maxner CE, Crawford S, Yuh WTC. Significance of CT and MR findings in sphenoid sinus disease. *AJNR* 1989;10:603–606.
43. Som PM, Dillon WP, Fullerton GD, Zimmerman RA, Rajagopalan B, Marom Z. Chronically obstructed sinonasal secretions: observations on T1 and T2 shortening. *Radiology* 1989;172:515–520.
44. Teresi L, Lufkin R, Hanafee W. Low cost MRI of the paranasal sinuses. *Comput Med Imaging Graph* 1988;12:165–168.
45. Trigaux JP, Berthand BM, Van Beers BE. Comparison of B-mode ultrasound, radiography and sinuscopy in the diagnosis of maxillary sinusitis. Report on 177 cases. *Acta Otorhinolaryngol Belg* 1988;42:670–679.
46. Shapiro GG, Furukawa CT, Pierson WE, Gilbertson E, Bierman CW. Blinded comparison of maxillary sinus radiograph and ultrasound for diagnosis of sinusitis. *J Allergy Clin Immunol* 1986;77:59–64.

47. Reilly JS, Hotaling AJ, Chiponis D, Wald ER. Use of ultrasound in detection of sinus disease in children. *Int J Pediatr Otorhinolaryngol* 1989;17:225–230.
48. Wald ER. Sinusitis in children. *Pediatr Infect Dis J* 1988;7:S150–S153.
49. Wald ER, Milmoe GJ, Bowen AD, Ledesma-Medina J, Salamon N, Bluestone CD. Acute maxillary sinusitis in children. *N Engl J Med* 1981;304:749–754.
50. Jannert M, Andreasson L, Helin I, Pettersson H. Acute sinusitis in children: symptoms, clinical findings and bacteriology related to initial radiologic appearance. *Int J Pediatr Otorhinolaryngol* 1982;4:139–148.
51. Dolan KD. Paranasal sinus radiology, part 1A: introduction and the frontal sinuses. *Head Neck Surg* 1982;4:301–311.
52. Wald ER. Management of sinusitis in infants and children. *Pediatr Infect Dis J* 1988;7:449–452.
53. Chakeres DW. Computed tomography of the ethmoid sinuses. *Otolaryngol Clin North Am* 1985;18:29–42.
54. Mancuso AA, Manafee WN. *Computed tomography and magnetic resonance imaging of the head and neck.* Baltimore: Williams & Wilkins, 1985;20–42.
55. Som PM, Lawson W, Biller HF, Lanzieri CF. Ethmoid sinus disease: CT evaluation in 400 cases. Part II. Postoperative findings. *Radiology* 1986;159:599–604.
56. Shapiro GG. The role of nasal airway obstruction in sinus disease and facial development. *J Allergy Clin Immunol* 1988;82:935–940.
57. Som PM. Paranasal sinuses and ptyerygopalatine fossa. In: Carter BL, ed. *Computed tomography of the head and neck,* vol 5 of *Contemporary issues in CT.* New York: Churchill Livingston, 1985;101–129.
58. Van Tassel PV, Lee Y-Y, Jing B-S, De Pena CA. Mucoceles of the paranasal sinuses: MR imaging with CT correlation. *AJR* 1989;153:407–412.
59. Som PM, Shugar JM. Antral mucoceles: a new look. *J Comput Assist Tomogr* 1980;4:484–488.
60. Hasso AN. CT of tumors and tumor-like conditions of the paranasal sinuses. *Radiol Clin North Am* 1984;22:119–130.
61. Centeno RS, Bentson JR, Mancuso AA. CT scanning in rhinocerebral mucormycosis and aspergillosis. *Radiology* 1981;140:383–389.
62. Lazo A, Wilner HI, Metes JJ. Craniofacial mucormycosis: computed tomographic and angiographic findings in two cases. *Radiology* 1981;139:623–626.
63. McGill TJ, Simpson G, Healy GB. Fulminant aspergillosis of the nose and paranasal sinuses: a new clinical entity. *Laryngoscope* 1980;90:748–754.
64. Gamba JL, Woodruff WW, Djang WT, Yeates AE. Craniofacial mucormyosis: assessment with CT. *Radiology* 1986;160:207–212.
65. Courey WR, New PFJ, Price DL. Angiographic manifestations of craniofacial mucormycosis. *Radiology* 1972;103:329–334.
66. Zinreich SJ, Kennedy DW, Malat J, et al. Fungal sinusitis: diagnosis with CT and MR imaging. *Radiology* 1988;169:439–444.
67. Manning SC, Vuitch F, Weinberg AG, Brown OE. Allergic aspergillosis: a newly recognized form of sinusitis in the pediatric population. *Laryngoscope* 1989;99:681–685.
68. Kopp W, Fotter R, Steiner H, Beaufort F, Stammberger H. Aspergillosis of the paranasal sinuses. *Radiology* 1985;156:715–716.
69. Silver AJ, Baredes S, Bello JA, Blitzer A, Hilal SK. The opacified maxillary sinus: CT findings in chronic sinusitis and malignant tumors. *Radiology* 1987;163:205–210.
70. Cuyler JP, Monaghan AJ. Cystic fibrosis and sinusitis. *J Otolaryngol* 1988;18:173–175.
71. Drake-Lee AB, Morgan DW. Nasal polyps and sinusitis in children with cystic fibrosis. *J Laryngol Otol* 1989;103:753–755.
72. Jaffe BF. Chronic sinusitis in children. *Clin Pediatr* 1974;13:944–948.
73. Hirsch M, Litshitz T. Computerized tomography in the diagnosis and treatment of orbital cellulitis. *Pediatr Radiol* 1988;18:302–305.
74. Wells RG, Sty JR, Gonnening RS. Imaging of the pediatric eye and orbit. *Radiographics* 1989;9:1023–1043.
75. Courville CB. Subdural empyema secondary to purulent frontal sinusitis. *Arch Otolaryngol* 1944;39:211–240.
76. Remmler D, Boles R. Intracranial complications of frontal sinusitis. *Laryngoscope* 1980;90:1814–1824.
77. Fairbanks DNF, Milmoe GJ. Complications and sequelae: an otolaryngologist's perspective. *Pediatr Infect Dis J* 1985;4:75–79.
78. Barkovich AJ. *Pediatric neuroimaging,* vol I, *Contemporary neuroimaging.* New York: Raven Press, 1990;293–326.
79. Maniglia AJ, Goodwin J, Arnold JE, Ganz E. Intracranial abscesses secondary to nasal, sinus, and orbital infections in adults and children. *Arch Otolaryngol Head Neck Surg* 1989;115:1424–1429.

Pediatric Sinusitis,
edited by R. P. Lusk,
Raven Press, Ltd., New York © 1992.

CHAPTER 4

Microbiology of Acute and Chronic Sinusitis

Ellen R. Wald

Despite the substantial prevalence and clinical importance of sinusitis of childhood, there has been relatively limited study of the microbiology of sinusitis in pediatric patients. In part this limitation is a reflection of the relative inaccessibility of the paranasal sinuses. Unlike the middle ear cavities, the paranasal sinuses cannot be directly inspected by the clinician. Furthermore, aspiration of the paranasal sinuses is not undertaken as easily and therefore not as often as tympanocentesis. This chapter reviews the published studies that have delineated the microbiology of acute and chronic sinusitis in children.

SINUS ASPIRATION

To determine the bacteriology of acute sinusitis, a sample of sinus secretions must be obtained from one of the paranasal sinuses without contamination by normal respiratory or oral flora that colonize mucosal surfaces. The maxillary sinus is the most accessible of the paranasal sinuses. A transnasal approach affords the easiest and safest route of sinus aspiration in pediatric patients. A trocar is passed beneath the inferior nasal turbinate across the lateral nasal wall. However, because the nasal vestibule is so heavily colonized, it is essential to attempt to sterilize the area of the nose beneath the inferior turbinate through which the trocar is passed. If this is not done, contaminating nasal flora isolated in the sinus aspirate may be misconstrued as pathogens. Sterilization can easily be accomplished with a topical solution of 4% cocaine. The advantage of cocaine versus povodine-iodine is that it provides both topical antisepsis and anesthesia and does not irritate the mucosa. Furthermore, to avoid misinterpre-

tation of culture results, infection is defined as the recovery of a bacterial species in high density, that is, a colony count of at least 10^4 colony forming units per milliliter (cfu/ml). This quantitative definition increases the probability that organisms recovered from the maxillary sinus aspirate truly represent *in situ* infection and not contamination. In fact, most sinus aspirates from infected sinuses are associated with colony counts in excess of 10^4 cfu/ml. If unable to perform quantitative cultures, Gram stain of aspirated specimens affords semiquantitative data. If bacteria are readily apparent on a Gram stain, the approximate bacterial density is 10^5 cfu/ml. The Gram stain can also be helpful in another way. If bacteria are seen on the smear of the specimen that fails to grow using standard aerobic culture techniques, anaerobic organisms or other fastidious bacteria should be suspected.

STUDY DESIGN

Using a study design similar to one described by investigators at the University of Virginia (1), we undertook an investigation of the microbiology of acute sinusitis in pediatric patients in 1979 (2). Patients were eligible for this study if they were between the ages of 2 and 16 years and presented with one of two clinical pictures—either onset with "persistent" or "severe" respiratory symptoms. The majority of subjects presented with "persistent" symptoms, that is, symptoms that lasted more than 10 but less than 30 days and had not yet begun to improve. A minimal duration of 10 days was used to separate simple upper respiratory infection (URI) from acute sinusitis and the maximum duration of 29 days was used to distinguish acute from subacute or chronic sinusitis. The time course of most simple URIs is 5 to 7 days. Although a patient with a URI may not be completely asymptomatic by the tenth day, he or she is almost always improved. Therefore

E. R. Wald: Department of Pediatrics, University of Pittsburgh School of Medicine, Children's Hospital of Pittsburgh, Pittsburgh, Pennsylvania 15213.

persistence of respiratory symptoms beyond 10 days, without improvement, suggests the presence of a bacterial complication, that is, sinusitis. The respiratory symptoms of acute sinusitis consist of nasal discharge of any quality (thick or thin, serous, mucoid, or purulent) or daytime cough or both. A smaller subset of subjects with acute sinusitis presented with "severe" respiratory symptoms. Severity was defined as high fever (temperature of at least 103°F) and purulent (thick, colored, and opaque) nasal discharge. For this presentation there was no qualifier on duration of symptoms. This clinical dyad is thought to signify sinus infection when contrasted with the course of the usual URI. Most simple URIs begin with clear nasal discharge, which may become purulent after a few days, but then reverts to a clear quality again before finally resolving. If fever is present at all during a URI, it usually occurs at the beginning of the viral syndrome. By the time the nasal discharge becomes purulent, most children with simple URIs are afebrile. Accordingly, the combination of purulent nasal discharge and fever is suggestive of a bacterial complication, that is, acute sinusitis.

Eligible children with either of these two presentations had sinus radiographs performed. The sinus films were considered to be abnormal if they showed diffuse opacification, mucosal thickening of greater than 4 mm, or an air–fluid level. If the sinus films were abnormal and informed consent was provided by the parent, then a sinus puncture was performed, using a transnasal approach.

MICROBIOLOGY OF ACUTE SINUSITIS

When a maxillary sinus aspirate was performed on children presenting with either persistent or severe symptoms and significantly abnormal sinus radiographs, bacteria in high density were recovered from 70% (3). Table 4.1 shows the bacterial species cultured from 79 sinus aspirates obtained from 50 children in their relative order of prevalence. *Streptococcus*

TABLE 4.1. *Bacterial species cultured from 79 sinus aspirates in 50 children*

Species	Single isolates	Multiple isolates	Total
Streptococcus pneumoniae	14	8	22
Moraxella catarrhalis	13	2	15
Hemophilus influenzae	10	5	15
Eikenella corrodens	1	0	1
Group A streptococcus	1	0	1
Group C streptococcus	0	1	1
Alpha-streptococcus	1	1	2
Peptostreptococcus	0	1	1
Moraxella spp	1	0	1

Adapted from ref. 3.

pneumoniae was most common, followed closely by *Branhamella catarrhalis* (now known as *Moraxella catarrhalis*), and *Hemophilus influenzae*. Both *M. catarrhalis* and *H. influenzae* may be beta-lactamase producing and thereby amoxicillin resistant. The *H. influenzae* found in sinus aspirates, like those found in infected middle ear cavities, are almost always the nontypeable organisms, reflecting their frequent colonization of the nasopharynx in contrast to *H. influenzae* type b. Only a single anaerobic bacterial species, *Peptostreptococcus*, was isolated. No staphylococci were recovered. Mixed infection with heavy growth of two bacterial species was occasionally found. In 25% of patients with bilateral maxillary sinusitis, there were discordant bacterial culture results. In some cases, one sinus aspirate was positive, while the other was negative. In the remaining cases, different bacterial species were recovered from each.

Viral cultures were also performed on the maxillary sinus aspirates. Since many children were evaluated after 10 or more days of symptoms, viruses were recovered infrequently. Adenovirus as the only isolate was grown from the aspirate of one subject; parainfluenza virus in combination with a bacterial isolate was recovered from a second (2). In studies of adults with acute sinusitis, other viruses including influenza and rhinovirus have been recovered from approximately 10% of sinus aspirates (1).

Recently, a study with nearly identical design was performed in Mexico City (4). Forty-four children ranging in age from 8 months to 12 years with upper respiratory symptoms of 1 to 4 weeks duration were evaluated. These children all had clinical and radiographic evidence of acute sinusitis. Maxillary sinus aspiration was performed as described in the previous study; specimens were cultured quantitatively. Aspirates were obtained from 84 sinuses from 44 children. Bacteria were recovered in colony counts of at least 10^4 cfu/ml from at least one sinus in 48% of subjects. *S. pneumoniae*, *H. influenzae*, and *Neisseria* species were most frequently isolated. The *Neisseria* species proved to be *N. subflava* rather than *Moraxella catarrhalis* when evaluated at the microbiology laboratory of the Children's Hospital of Pittsburgh.

MICROBIOLOGY OF SUBACUTE SINUSITIS

We recently summarized our experience with children having subacute sinusitis (5). These youngsters were evaluated in the context of several different comparative trials of antimicrobial therapy. All children had persistent respiratory symptoms—nasal discharge or cough or both lasting between 30 and 120 days. These children were generally well (with minimal constitutional complaints) except for their respiratory

TABLE 4.2. *Bacterial species cultured from 52 sinus aspirates in 40 children*

Species	Single isolates	Multiple isolates	Total
Streptococcus pneumoniae	9	3	12
Hemophilus influenzae	9	2	11
Moraxella catarrhalis	6	2	8
Streptococcus pyogenes	2	0	2
Streptococcus viridans	0	1	1
Moraxella species	0	1	1

Adapted from ref. 5.

symptoms. Intermittent fever was a complaint in 25% of patients but was rarely documented at the time of presentation. Some of these children had previously received one or more courses of antimicrobial agents. In each case they either failed to respond to the antimicrobial or improved only slightly and experienced symptomatic recurrence following cessation of antibiotics. Table 4.2 shows the bacterial species cultured from 52 sinus aspirates from 40 children. Again, the three predominant organisms were *S. pneumoniae*, *H. influenzae*, and *M. catarrhalis*.

MICROBIOLOGY OF CHRONIC SINUSITIS

Chronic sinusitis has received only limited study in pediatric patients. In 1981, Brook (6) published a study in which he evaluated 40 pediatric patients with what he described as chronic sinusitis. He defined chronic sinusitis as respiratory symptoms that lasted more than 3 weeks. Some of his subjects had underlying disorders including allergic conditions in twelve, local intranasal problems in five, and cystic fibrosis in one. In 50% of these patients, specimens for culture were obtained at the time of sinus surgery. Presumably these patients had more protracted and more severe disease than the patients we have discussed thus far. Table 4.3 shows the bacteria isolated from 37 of these 40 patients. Anaerobes were isolated from all these patients. The most common organisms were anaerobic gram-positive cocci such as staphylococci and streptococci. Another large group was the *Bacteroides* species, especially *Bacteroides melaninogenicus*. Fusobacteria were also recovered often. Aerobes were isolated in approximately 38%. The most common aerobes were streptococci and staphylococci. *Hemophilus* species were isolated from only four patients.

Quantitative cultures of sinus secretions were not performed in Brook's study. For specimens obtained at surgery this omission probably did not result in the introduction of potentially confounding mucosal contamination because of better sterile technique. However, as previously discussed, the lack of quantitation when culturing sinus aspirates may lead to ambiguous results. In Brook's study, aspirates may have been performed in as many as 50% of patients. Note, for example, that *Propionibacterium acnes* was recovered from eight patients. This bacterial isolate is usual skin

TABLE 4.3. *Bacteria isolated from 37 children with chronic sinusitis*

Isolates Aerobic and facultative	Number of isolates	Isolates Anaerobic	Number of isolates
Gram-positive cocci		Anaerobic cocci	
Alpha-hemolytic streptococci	7	*Peptococcus* species	14
Group A beta-hemolytic streptococci	3	*Peptostreptococcus* species	6
Group F beta-hemolytic streptococci	1	*Streptococcus constelatus*	1
Staphylococcus aureus	7	Microaerophilic streptococci	7
Staphylococcus epidermidis	1	*Veillonella parvula*	6
Gram-negative bacilli		Gram-positive bacilli	
Escherichia coli	1	*Eubacterium* species	2
Hemophilus influenzae	2	*Propionibacterium acnes*	8
Hemophilus parainfluenzae	2	*Propionibacterium avidum*	1
Total	24	*Clostridium* species	3
		Gram-negative bacilli	
		Fusobacterium species	6
		F. nucleatum	5
		F. mortiferum	1
		F. necrophorum	1
		Bacteroides species	10
		B. melaninogenicus	14
		B. oralis	5
		B. ruminicola ss brevis	5
		B. corrodens	1
		B. biacutus	1
		Total	97

Adapted from ref. 6.

or nasal flora and its recovery in low density almost certainly denotes contamination.

Muntz and Lusk (7) recently reported the bacteriology of the ethmoid bullae in 105 children between the ages of 9 months and 17 years with chronic sinusitis. Specimens for culture were obtained from the mucosa of the anterior ethmoid cell in patients undergoing endoscopic ethmoidectomy. All had received at least two courses of an appropriate antimicrobial and were treated until the day before surgery. Although nasal decongestion was achieved with topical cocaine, contamination of the residual ethmoid flora by nasal flora may not be completely avoidable. Furthermore, no quantitation of the bacterial isolates was performed and antibiotics may surely have eradicated or prevented the growth of other bacterial flora. The most common bacterial species to be recovered were alpha-hemolytic streptococci and *Staphylococcus aureus* followed by *S. pneumoniae*, *H. influenzae*, and *M. catarrhalis*. Anaerobic organisms were grown from 6% of specimens. This report details the residual bacterial flora in patients treated for chronic sinusitis with antimicrobials effective against beta-lactamase producing bacterial species.

The report of data concerning pediatric patients with chronic sinusitis by Tinkleman and Silk (8) is mentioned in the interest of completeness despite its many and substantial methodologic problems. The study relates bacteriologic findings in 35 of 116 children evaluated for sinusitis at four different hospitals. Standardization of technique is quite unlikely, as evidenced by the fact that culture and sensitivity results were not obtained on 77 patients. Furthermore, all patients were on antibiotics at the time of their surgical procedures. The predominant bacterial isolates were *H. influenzae*,

S. pneumoniae, and *M. catarrhalis*. Group A streptococcus and *S. aureus* were isolated from three patients each.

Another report of patients with probable chronic sinusitis was that of Shapiro et al. (9), who studied 20 patients with cystic fibrosis. In these patients with chronic cough and paranasal sinuses that are nearly uniformly opacified on x-ray, a clinical diagnosis of sinusitis may be difficult to make. Patients were enrolled when they had increased respiratory symptoms—especially nasal discharge and exacerbations of cough. Maxillary sinus aspirates and quantitative cultures were performed as described previously (1). Table 4.4 shows the bacterial etiology of sinusitis in these patients. The most common aerobes identified were *Pseudomonas aeruginosa*, *H. influenzae*, and alpha-hemolytic streptococci. The anaerobes recovered included anaerobic streptococci, *Bacteroides oralis*, *P. acnes*, and one unidentified gram-negative rod.

MICROBIOLOGY OF SINUSITIS IN ASTHMATIC CHILDREN

There have been several very small studies of asthmatic children with sinusitis. These are probably best presented with the chronic sinusitis group as many patients may be experiencing acute exacerbations of a chronic mucosal process. One such study of eight patients was reported in 1984 (10). Sinus puncture and quantitation were performed as described (2). In this small study, half the children had positive maxillary sinus aspirates. The bacterial species recovered included *M. catarrhalis*, *H. influenzae*, and *S. pneumoniae*. A more recent investigation evaluating 12 children between 3 and 11 years of age with asthma was reported by Goldenhersh et al. (11). In this study all subjects had documented respiratory allergy and chronic respiratory symptoms of at least 30 days duration consistent with chronic sinusitis. All patients had opacification of one or both maxillary sinuses. When maxillary sinus aspiration was performed, *M. catarrhalis* was recovered from six patients and mixed cultures of streptococci were recovered from three patients. Only one patient had anaerobic streptococci mixed with aerobic streptococci.

CONCLUSION

The studies reviewed in this chapter, excepting those reported by Brook (6) and Shapiro et al. (8), have shown remarkably consistent results regarding the microbiology of sinusitis in children. The exceptional bacteriology of sinus infection in patients with cystic fibrosis is not surprising. However, Brook's results

TABLE 4.4. *Bacteria recovered from aspirate material from the maxillary sinuses of 20 patients with cystic fibrosis*

Bacteria	Number of sinuses	Only organism isolated
Aerobes	30	—
Pseudomonas aeruginosa	13	7
Hemophilus influenzae	10	5
Nontypeable	9	4
Type A	1	1
Alpha-hemolytic streptococci (including microaerophilic streptococci)	5	3
Escherichia coli	1	1
Staphylococcus aureus	1	1
Anaerobes	5	—
Peptostreptococcus species	2	—
Bacteroides oralis	1	—
Propionibacterium acnes	1	—
Unidentified gram-negative rod	1	1

Adapted from ref. 7.

can only be reconciled with the rest by allowing that his patients are different from those studied by other investigators, either in the duration or severity of their symptoms.

The microbiology associated with sinusitis can be anticipated according to the patterns of clinical presentation. In patients with acute, subacute, or chronic sinusitis who are generally well except for persistent respiratory symptoms, the usual bacterial isolates are *S. pneumoniae, H. influenzae*, and *M. catarrhalis*. In contrast, anaerobic organisms and staphylococci should be suspected in patients with very long-standing symptoms or in those whose symptoms are so severe or complicated that sinus surgery is undertaken. Alpha-hemolytic streptococci other than pneumococci become important in patients with protracted symptoms.

REFERENCES

1. Evans RD Jr, Sydnor JB, Moore WEC, et al. Sinusitis of the maxillary antrum. *N Engl J Med* 1975;293:735–739.
2. Wald ER, Milmoe GJ, Bowen AD, Ledesma-Medina J, Salmon N, Bluestone CD. Acute maxillary sinusitis in children. *N Engl J Med* 1981;304:749–754.
3. Wald ER, Reilly JS, Casselbrant M, et al. Treatment of acute maxillary sinusitis in childhood: a comparative study of amoxicillin and cefaclor. *J Pediatr* 1984;104:297–302.
4. Rodriguez RS, De La Torre C, Sanchez C, et al. Bacteriology and treatment of acute maxillary sinusitis in children: a comparative study of erythromycin-sulfisoxazole and amoxicillin. Abstracts of the Interscience Conference of Antimicrobial Agents and Chemotherapy (328), Los Angeles, 1988.
5. Wald ER, Byers C, Guerra N, Casselbrant M, Beste D. Subacute sinusitis in children. *J Pediatr* 1989;115:28–32.
6. Brook I. Bacteriologic features of chronic sinusitis in children. *JAMA* 1981;246:967–969.
7. Muntz HR, Lusk RP. Bacteriology of the ethmoid bullae in children with chronic sinusitis. *Arch Otolaryngol Head Neck Surg* 1991;117:179–181.
8. Tinkleman DG, Silk HJ. Clinical and bacteriologic features of chronic sinusitis in children. *Am J Dis Child* 1989;143:938–941.
9. Shapiro ED, Milmoe GJ, Wald ER, Rodnan JB, Bowen AD. Bacteriology of the maxillary sinuses in patients with cystic fibrosis. *J Infect Dis* 1982;146:589–593.
10. Friedman R, Ackerman W, Wald E, Casselbrant M, Friday G, Fireman P. Asthma and bacterial sinusitis in children. *J Allergy Clin Immunol* 1984;74:185–189.
11. Goldenhersh MJ, Rachelefsky GS, Dudley J, et al. The bacteriology of chronic maxillary sinusitis in children with respiratory allergy. *J Allergy Clin Immunol* 1990;85:1030–1039.

Pediatric Sinusitis,
edited by R. P. Lusk,
Raven Press, Ltd., New York © 1992.

CHAPTER 5

Sinusitis and Allergy

Gail G. Shapiro

Quite often the physical examination of the child with a history of sinus disease reveals boggy mucosa. The inference is made that this sort of environment might well occlude ostia and disturb normal clearance mechanisms, thereby predisposing the patient to infection. Naturally, on seeing swollen, congested mucosa, one thinks of allergy. Allergic rhinitis is probably the most common cause of chronic nasal congestion in children, and allergic disease affects 15 to 20% of the U.S. population.

PATHOPHYSIOLOGY OF ALLERGIC RHINITIS

Allergic rhinitis results from an IgE-mediated reaction of the nasal membranes. Mucosal mast cells and basophils of individuals who are allergic to inhaled allergens such as dust mites and pollens are coated with immunoglobulin E directed toward epitopes of these foreign molecules. While the F_c portion of the IgE molecules are fixed to the cells, the Fab portions offer the binding sites for the allergens. The bridging of two IgE molecules by allergen results in cellular changes that allow allergic mediator release. Preformed mediators such as histamine are released within minutes. Some of these mediators recruit inflammatory cells to the site of the allergic reactions; some appear to influence basophils to secrete allergic mediators hours after the initial antigen–immunoglobulin E union (Fig. 5.1).

While the role of each currently identifiable mediator has not been clarified, the overall effect is vascular dilatation, mucosal edema, and mucus hypersecretion through the direct effect of mediators like histamine on vascular integrity as well as reflex stimulation of mucosal glands through nerve endings in the mucosa and submucosa. The resulting structural disruption advances the ability of antigen to further enter the environment and perpetuate the allergic reaction (1,2).

CLINICAL OBSERVATIONS CONNECTING ALLERGIC RHINITIS AND SINUSITIS

While observations connecting allergy and sinusitis can be traced back through time, there is a renaissance of interest and literature on the subject dating from the late 1970s (Table 5.1). At that time, during a 1-year period in Seattle, we evaluated a large number of children who presented for workup of possible allergic disease and who had similar and distinctive signs and symptoms that suggested problems besides allergic diathesis (3). In all, there were 91 children with persistent cough, chronic rhinorrhea, fatigue, and irritability who did not benefit from typical allergy-directed therapy (e.g., antihistamines and decongestants) from their primary care physician. Cough was often the primary complaint, with many parents complaining of their children's sleepless nights due to cough. Typically, on physical examination, patients showed nasal edema often with purulent rhinorrhea or posterior pharyngeal drainage. A large portion also had evidence of coexisting ear problems: effusion, marked negative middle ear pressure, or ventilating tubes verifying previous ear disease. Nasal cytology was obtained by having patients blow their noses into plastic wrap. The secretions were applied to glass slides and processed with Hansel's stain. The smears showed a predominance of polymorphonuclear neutrophils with intracellular bacteria in most patients. Nasal eosinophilia, typical of allergic disease, was notably absent. Sinus radiographs (Waters view) showed marked membrane thickening (> 6 mm) or opacification of one or both maxillary antra in 64 patients, 70% of the sample. While the therapeutic trial was not controlled, a reg-

G. G. Shapiro: University of Washington School of Medicine, and Northwest Asthma & Allergy Center, Seattle, Washington 98105.

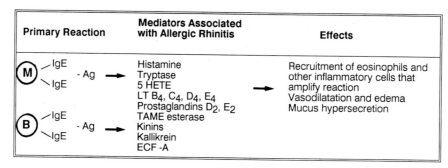

Primary Reaction	Mediators Associated with Allergic Rhinitis	Effects
(M) IgE — Ag → IgE	Histamine Tryptase 5 HETE LT B$_4$, C$_4$, D$_4$, E$_4$ Prostaglandins D$_2$, E$_2$	Recruitment of eosinophils and other inflammatory cells that amplify reaction Vasodilatation and edema Mucus hypersecretion
(B) IgE — Ag → IgE	TAME esterase Kinins Kallikrein ECF -A	

FIG. 5.1. This schematic diagram is a simplified summary of the major events that produce symptomatic allergic rhinitis. M, mast cell; B, basophil; IgE, Immunoglobulin E; Ag, antigen; LT, leukotriene; ECF-A, eosinophil chemotactic factor of anaphylaxis; HETE, hydroxyeicosatetraenoic acid; TAME, tosyl.

imen of amoxicillin, oral antihistamine–decongestant, and short-term use of a vasoconstrictor nose spray appeared to lead to improvement in most cases, with disappearance of cough, rhinorrhea, and other complaints. In many subjects, along with clinical improvement the nasal secretions changed so that there were few neutrophils, few bacteria, and increased likelihood of eosinophilia.

A parallel evaluation occurred at the same time in Los Angeles, again in an allergy practice. In a prospective manner, Rachelefsky and co-workers (4) evaluated 70 children referred to their allergy practice for chronic respiratory symptoms. They included sinus radiography and nasal cytology in this assessment. They cited the most important finding in this study as the high prevalence of abnormal sinus radiographs in this population of allergic children, 37 subjects (53%) having some abnormality with 15 (21%) having complete opacification of one or both maxillary antra. The patients with marked radiographic abnormalities tended to be younger (mean age 6.5 years versus 9.2 for the unaffected group) and had more impressive histories of rhinorrhea and cough. The nasal smear with neutrophils and low number of eosinophils was the only helpful laboratory test suggesting sinus disease. The majority of patients with sinus involvement responded favorably to a 2-week course of ampicillin and pseudoephedrine and a short course of oxymetazoline nose spray. Several patients failed to improve even after additional medical therapy and required maxillary antral puncture, which yielded purulent material.

These two evaluations have remarkable similarities. In both cases children presenting for evaluation of res-

TABLE 5.1. *Clinical observations connecting allergic rhinitis and sinusitis*

Shapiro	Ref. 3
Rachelefsky et al.	Ref. 4
Lehrer et al.	Ref. 5
Shapiro et al.	Ref. 6

piratory allergy had a high incidence of sinus disease. At the time of these observations, it was the sinus disease rather than allergy that was the focus of attention. Now in the 1990s it is impossible in retrospect to ascertain the actual incidence of significant allergic disease among these patients. While many were, indeed, atopic individuals, it is likely that a portion were not allergic but were chronically symptomatic due to untreated or undertreated sinusitis.

Looking at the situation differently, Lehrer and co-workers (5) presented a preliminary report in 1981 of 14 patients presenting with recurrent tonsillitis, pharyngitis, and sinusitis who had significantly elevated total serum IgE and/or specific IgE to common inhalant allergens measured by *in vitro* assay (modified RAST). After a year of allergic immunotherapy, the incidence of infection was markedly reduced and surgery was usually averted. It is not clear how many patients were seen who had the same diseases but were not allergic. Also, it is unclear whether other factors besides immunotherapy might have affected outcome, such as better medical management of infectious episodes. The authors acknowledge the weakness of such a retrospective evaluation but believe that the importance of underlying allergy in the pathogenesis of upper respiratory infections is major.

Focusing on chronic and difficult to manage sinusitis, Shapiro and co-workers (6) evaluated 61 children and adolescents with at least 6 months of refractory sinusitis, that is, patients requiring repeated courses of appropriate antibiotics, some of whom finally required surgical intervention. In these patients, they assessed quantitative immunoglobulins including IgG subclasses as well as immune response to *H. influenzae* and pneumococcal vaccines. They also noted the allergic status of the patients in terms of highest degree of responsiveness to inhalant skin tests and incidence of elevated serum IgE concentration. Twenty-two patients had prick test reactivity, 12 had intense intradermal test reactivity (wheal 5 mm larger than in saline control, also with pseudopods), and 21 had some intradermal reactivity, possibly significant (wheal 5 mm larger than in saline control without pseudopods). Five patients had serum IgE over two standard deviations of that predicted for age, and three of these were also prick test responders. Combining those patients with high total IgE or marked skin test reactivity yields 36 of 61 or almost 60% of the sample, much higher than the 15 to 20% incidence of allergy in the general population. One does not know, unfortunately, whether this is skewed upward by referral preselection to the investigators' allergy/immunology practice.

IMAGING STUDIES CONNECTING ALLERGY AND SINUSITIS

Imaging techniques offer some insight into the relationship between sinusitis and allergy. Slavin and co-workers (7) presented a pilot study suggesting that there might be such an entity as allergic sinusitis. They evaluated three patients with ragweed allergic rhinitis using single photon emission computerized tomography (SPEC). This technique indicated hyperemia and increased metabolic activity in the paranasal sinuses even though radiographs were normal.

Pelikan and Pelikan-Filipek (8) published an intriguing evaluation of the relationship between nasal antigen challenge and changes in sinus radiographs. Thirty-seven patients with chronic maxillary sinusitis were exposed to nasal provocation tests with a variety of inhalant allergens. Twenty-nine patients developed 41 positive challenges. Of the 41, 32 positive challenges (78%) were associated with changes on sinus radiographs, changes including increased mucosal edema or opacification. Often symptoms including pressure in the maxillary area, acute headache, and otalgia accompanied the changes. In contrast, only 2 of 11 negative challenges (18%) were associated with distinct changes on radiograph. All positive nasal challenges were accompanied by acute nasal symptoms such as blockage, hypersecretion, sneezing, and itching.

TABLE 5.2. *Survey of nasal response (NRs) and sinus maxillaris response (SMRs) after nasal challenge with allergen*

Patients N = 37	Positive NRs		Negative NRs	
	SMRs +	SMRs +	SMRs −	SMRs −
29 Patients with 41 Positive NRs	32	9		
11 Negative NRs			2	9
8 Patients with 21 Negative NRs			3	18
37 Control PBS challenges	0	0	0	37

From ref. 8, with permission.

Among 37 control challenges with buffered saline, there were no changes on sinus radiographs and no nasal symptoms (Table 5.2).

THE EOSINOPHIL AND SINUSITIS

The eosinophil appears to be a culprit in sinusitis just as it is in the inflammatory changes of asthma. The proclivity of eosinophils of allergic individuals to reside in nasal and probably sinus mucosa suggests that there will be a likely environment for the sort of destructive changes that eosinophils can induce. Harlin et al. (9) demonstrated a chronic eosinophilic infiltration in sinus mucosa of patients with chronic sinusitis, both those with and without nasal allergy, and underscored the toxic potential of the eosinophil.

Recently, Hisamatsu and co-workers (10) demonstrated the toxic effects of human eosinophil granule major basic protein (MBP) on nasal mucosa *in vitro*. Both changes in the mucosal surface and ciliary activity were inhibited within hours of exposure. Interestingly, mucosa from allergic patients was damaged by concentrations of MBP that had no effect on mucosal specimens from a normal individual. This reinforces that the allergic patient may be at higher risk of sinus disease because of the known association of eosinophilia and allergy; that is, being an allergic person makes you more likely to harbor nasal eosinophils, which have toxic potential. In addition, allergic patients may have mucosal vulnerability that is beyond the normal patient's. Both of these situations would predispose the allergic patient to sinus disease.

CONCLUSIONS

While these interesting associations between sinusitis, allergy, and eosinophilic mucosal disease suggest a meaningful connection, there is still no firm proof of a cause and effect relationship. Thus far, no controlled observation of incidence of sinusitis among allergic versus nonallergic patients has been carried out. To do this, one would need to clearly define allergic and nonallergic criteria as well as criteria for diagnosing sinusitis. Patients would need to be matched for age and environmental factors, leaving allergic status as the only major difference between the groups. Then these samples would need to be followed prospectively. Until this is done, we are left with the possibility of an association between allergy and sinusitis that is based on the likelihood that nasal airway obstruction secondary to allergic rhinitis results in membrane edema, mucus hypersecretion, eosinophil-induced destruction, and subsequent ostial obstruction and mucus stasis, which might well predispose to inflammatory changes in the sinus and to infection.

REFERENCES

1. Howarth PH, Holgate ST. Basic aspects of allergic reactions. In: Naspitz CK, Tinkelman DG, eds. *Childhood rhinitis and sinusitis*. New York: Marcel Dekker, 1990;2–37.
2. Flowers BK, Naclerio RM. The nose. In: Naspitz CK, Tinkelman DG, eds. *Childhood rhinitis and sinusitis*. New York: Marcel Dekker, 1990;147–192.
3. Shapiro GG. Role of allergy in sinusitis. *Pediatr Infect Dis* 1985;4(6):55–58.
4. Rachelefsky GS, Goldberg M, Katz RM, et al. Sinus disease in children with respiratory allergy. *J Allergy Clin Immunol* 1978;61(5):310–314.
5. Lehrer JF, Ali M, Silver J, Cordes B. Recognition and treatment of allergy in sinusitis and pharyngotonsillitis. *Arch Otolaryngol* 1981;107:543–546.
6. Shapiro GG, Virant FS, Furukawa CT, Pierson WE, Bierman CW. Immunologic defects in patients with refractory sinusitis. *Pediatrics* 1991;87:311–316.
7. Slavin RG, et al. Is there such an entity as allergic sinusitis? *J Allergy Clin Immunol* 1988;81:284 (abstract).
8. Pelikan Z, Pelikan-Filipek M. Role of nasal allergy in chronic sinusitis maxillaris (CSM)—diagnostic value of nasal challenge with allergen (NPT). *J Allergy Clin Immunol* 1990;86:484–491.
9. Harlin SL, Ansel DG, Lane SR, Myers J, Kephart GM, Gleich GJ. A clinical and pathologic study of chronic sinusitis: the role of the eosinophil. *J Allergy Clin Immunol* 1988;81:867–875.
10. Hisamatsu K, Ganbo T, Nakazawa T, Murakami Y, Gleich GJ, Makiyama K, Koyama H. Cytotoxicity of human eosinophil granule major basic protein to human nasal sinus mucosa *in vitro*. *J Allergy Clin Immunol* 1990;86:52–63.

Pediatric Sinusitis,
edited by R. P. Lusk,
Raven Press, Ltd., New York © 1992.

CHAPTER 6

Sinusitis and Immune Deficiency

Stephen H. Polmar

Sinusitis is a common illness in children. The last decade has witnessed a growing awareness of the magnitude of this problem by pediatricians, allergists, and otolaryngologists (1–4). Respiratory allergy has been recognized as a major factor that predisposes children to recurrent and chronic sinusitis (1,5). Allergic children with symptoms of rhinitis and/or asthma have a high frequency of sinusitis (5,6). As in adults, sinusitis has been shown to be an aggravating factor in both atopic and nonatopic children with asthma (6). However, not all children with recurrent/chronic sinusitis who were initially thought to be allergic are found to be so after allergy evaluation. Within this group of patients, one may identify children with immunodeficiency diseases, ciliary immotility disorders, and cystic fibrosis (4). In this chapter we restrict discussion to the recognition of immunodeficiency disease in the sinusitis-prone child and its implications for therapy. For a review of general principles of immunology and detailed descriptions of childhood primary immunodeficiency diseases, the reader is referred to refs. 7–9.

RECOGNITION OF IMMUNODEFICIENCY IN THE SINUSITIS-PRONE CHILD

The immunodeficient child will suffer recurrent and/or chronic sinusitis. Thus immunodeficiency should not be sought in the patient who only suffers an occasional bout of acute sinusitis. A child should be designated as "sinusitis-prone" if he/she suffers three or more episodes of sinusitis within a year or if he/she requires antibiotic therapy for control of sinusitis for 3 or more months during a year. The majority of sinusitis-prone children are atopic rather than immunodeficient. Respiratory allergy occurs in 8 to 20% of children while estimates of the incidence of all immunodeficiency diseases of childhood combined are less than 0.5% (7). Therefore, solely on the basis of odds, it is 16- to 40-fold more likely to detect allergy in a sinusitis-prone child than it is to find immunodeficiency. These calculations would apply to a primary care practice. In specialty practices and regional referral centers, the frequency of immunodeficient patients is likely to be higher. Recently, Shapiro and coworkers (10) reported immunologic defects in approximately one-third of the children with refractory sinusitis referred to their practice by pediatricians and family practitioners for suspected allergy.

The symptoms of sinusitis in the immunodeficient child are the same as in the allergic or immunologically normal child. Nasal obstruction, nasal discharge, and day- and night-coughing are the predominant symptoms. Sore throat, postnasal drip, halitosis, malaise, fatigue, and irritability occur frequently, while headache and fever are rare. Thus one cannot identify the immunodeficient patient on the basis of the severity or other characteristics of the sinusitis episode. Middle ear disease occurs in high frequency in both allergic patients (4) and immunodeficient children (11) who are sinusitis-prone. Recurrent otitis media with effusion often precedes the appearance of sinusitis in both groups. Other characteristics may, however, assist in discriminating the allergic patient from the immunodeficient one. The allergic patient is likely to have a family history of allergy, a seasonal pattern of respiratory symptoms, and a favorable response to antihistamines. Nasal pruritis, itching eyes, wheezing, eczema, and food allergy are more commonly associated with allergy than with immunodeficiency, although exceptions do exist. The occurrence of frequent bacterial infections in addition to respiratory tract infections should alert the physician to the pos-

S. H. Polmar: Washington University School of Medicine, and St. Louis Children's Hospital, St. Louis, Missouri 63110.

sibility of immunodeficiency. The undiagnosed immunodeficient child is virtually always taking an antibiotic and becomes ill shortly after antibiotics are discontinued. Recurrent pneumonias, meningitis, cellulitis, oral and/or cutaneous candidiasis, chronic diarrhea, and failure to thrive are hallmarks of some of the more severe childhood immunodeficiency disorders (7,8). However, in the most common immune deficiency diseases, recurrent/chronic sinusitis, with or without otitis media, may be the only indication that a patient is immunodeficient. Since many immunodeficiency diseases are hereditary, the presence of a positive family history for immunodeficiency or other individuals with recurrent infections is also helpful in recognizing the immunodeficient patient.

The recognition of the immunodeficient patient from within the group of sinusitis-prone children is based primarily on history and, to a lesser extent, physical examination. Laboratory studies should be considered confirmatory and should not be used for "screening" or in lieu of a careful history. No one laboratory test will detect all immunodeficient patients.

SPECTRUM OF IMMUNODEFICIENCY DISEASES IN SINUSITIS-PRONE CHILDREN

Immunodeficient children who come to clinical attention because of recurrent/chronic sinusitis have primarily humoral immunodeficiency diseases. These include immunoglobulin deficiency, selective IgG subclass deficiency, selective antibody deficiency, and complement component deficiency. Patients with defects in T-lymphocyte function such as those with severe combined immunodeficiency disease or neutrophil dysfunction (e.g., chronic granulomatous disease) will usually present with more severe infections and if sinusitis is present, it is not a prominent problem. While sinusitis may occur in HIV-infected patients, it is rarely the reason they come to clinical attention. Fungal sinusitis occurs rarely in children. In these instances impairment of neutrophil-, macrophage-, and/or T-lymphocyte function should be considered.

Deficiencies of immunoglobulin and/or antibody production are the most common immune defects and also comprise the majority of the immunodeficient patients who are sinusitis-prone. Table 6.1 lists the frequency of various immunodeficiency diseases seen in sinusitis-prone patients in our pediatric immunology clinic.

Common Variable Immunodeficiency (CVID)

Recurrent/chronic sinusitis is the most common clinical presentation of CVID patients. CVID is a disorder in which patients have significantly reduced levels of

TABLE 6.1. *Frequency of various immunodeficiency diseases among sinusitis-prone immunodeficient patients seen in the Washington University Pediatric Immunology Clinic*

Diagnosis	Number of patients
Common variable immunodeficiency	9
IgG-subclass deficiency	8
Selective antibody deficiency	6
IgA deficiency	5
C4 deficiency	3
X-linked agammaglobulinemia	1
Ataxia-telangiectasia	1
Hyper-IgM immunodeficiency	1

two or more immunoglobulin classes (usually IgG and IgA) in serum and are unable to synthesize antibodies to antigens which they have not previously encountered. IgG levels are generally less than 200 mg/dl; IgA and IgM are usually low as well. Response to primary immunization is poor, and retention of antibody from previous immunizations is variable. Onset of infections varies from 2 years of age through adulthood. These patients also suffer recurrent otitis media, bronchitis, and pneumonias; however, some may have sinusitis as their only recurrent or chronic infection. CVID is highly variable as its name implies. Most CVID patients have normal or near-normal numbers of B-lymphocytes in contrast to patients with X-linked agammaglobulinemia. CVID is familial but does not follow a classical mendelian pattern of inheritance.

IgG Subclass Deficiency

IgG comprises four subclasses: IgG1, IgG2, IgG3, and IgG4. IgG1 makes up approximately 60 to 70% of total serum IgG, IgG2 20%, IgG3 10%, and IgG4 less than 5%. Thus one may have a significant deficiency of one or more IgG subclasses and still have a normal or near-normal level of total IgG. The most common selective IgG-subclass deficiency in children is IgG2 deficiency (12,13). IgG2 or IgG2–IgG4 deficiency frequently occurs in association with IgA deficiency as well as in ataxia-telangiectasia (14,15). Some IgG2-deficient patients are unable to synthesize antibodies when immunized with the polysaccharides of *Hemophilus influenzae* or *Streptococcus pneumoniae* (16). IgG3 is the most common subclass deficiency in adults but occurs in children as well. Many antiviral antibodies are of the IgG3 subclass but IgG3-deficient patients seem to be able to make antiviral antibodies normally. Selective IgG1 deficiency is rare and selective IgG4 deficiency has been reported, but its clinical significance remains unclear. Recurrent/chronic sinusitis, otitis media, bronchitis, reactive airway disease, and pneumonia are the most characteristic clinical features of IgG-subclass-deficient patients. The natural history of IgG-subclass deficiency in children is not completely understood. In some children subclass deficiency is transient (17). This was suspected because IgG2 deficiency, which occurs in approximately one-half of all subclass-deficient children, occurs in only 7% of subclass-deficient adults (13). Alternatively, we have observed patients with subclass deficiency progress to CVID. In other patients it is likely that the subclass deficiency will persist unchanged.

Selective Antibody Deficiency

Patients may suffer recurrent infections because of inability to produce specific antibodies to a limited number of antigens. Most commonly, patients are unable to synthesize protective levels of antibody to pneumococcal polysaccharides but readily produce antibody to protein antigens such as diphtheria- and tetanus toxoids as well as to viral coat proteins. Selective antibody deficiency may occur in patients with normal immunoglobulin levels (18) or in those with a selective IgG-subclass deficiency (16). In a recent study of children with refractory sinusitis, approximately one-third of the patients failed to respond to one or more pneumococcal polysaccharide types, with poor response to type 7 polysaccharide being the most frequently observed abnormality (10). In the same study only 5% of patients failed to make antibody to *H. influenzae* type B polysaccharide vaccine. It should be noted that children rarely respond to immunization with purified polysaccharide vaccines prior to the age of 2 years and responses to some types (pneumococcal types 9 and 14) are normally poor in children. Pneumococcal polysaccharide types 3 and 7 are most helpful in detected selective antibody deficiencies. In the same study (10), the majority of patients with selective antipneumococcal antibody deficiency had normal serum immunoglobulin and IgG-subclass levels. It is not known whether selective antibody deficiency in children such as these will be permanent or transient.

IgA Deficiency

Selective IgA deficiency occurs in up to 0.2% of the adult population. In children IgA levels rise relatively slowly and the diagnosis of selective IgA deficiency (serum IgA less than 5 mg/dl) cannot be made reliably before 2 years of age. Some patients with apparent selective IgA deficiency have an increased susceptibility to respiratory tract infection including recurrent sinusitis. However, other IgA-deficient individuals show no increased susceptibility to infection. Patients with IgA deficiency associated with IgG2- or IgG2–IgG4-subclass deficiency appear to be more susceptible to respiratory tract infections than those who do not have associated subclass deficiencies (14). We have observed that some patients with selective IgA deficiency who are sinusitis-prone have an associated selective inability to synthesize antibodies to pneumococcal polysaccharides. In children under 6 years of age IgA deficiency may be transient.

X-Linked Agammaglobulinemia (XLA)

Patients with XLA are severely deficient in IgG, IgM, IgA, and IgE as well as IgG subclasses and are unable to synthesize antibodies to virtually any antigen. They lack B-cells in their blood, and plasma cells are absent from bone marrow, mucous membranes, and lymph nodes; peripheral lymphoid tissues (lymph nodes and tonsils) are decreased in size. These patients manifest an increased susceptibility to infection, particularly with pyogenic bacteria, beginning at 6 to 12 months of age. Patients frequently experience severe systemic bacterial infections such as pneumonia, meningitis, septic arthritis, cellulitis, and septicemia. Recurrent otitis media and sinusitis also occur. Immunoglobulin replacement with intravenous immunoglobulin (IVIG) is definitely indicated for these patients and virtually eliminates their susceptibility to severe infections. In our experience, most patients with XLA receiving adequate amounts of IVIG (see below) only occasionally suffer sinusitis.

Complement Component Deficiency

Deficiencies of serum complement components are a relatively rare cause of recurrent/chronic sinusitis. Overall, complement component deficiencies comprise only 2% of all immunodeficiency diseases. In our clinic we found three sinusitis-prone children with persistent deficiency (less than 15 mg/dl) of the C4 component of complement. Patients with C4B deficiency have been found to have an increased susceptibility to meningitis (19). Other complement component deficiencies have not been reported to be associated with recurrent/chronic sinusitis.

Other Immunodeficiency Diseases

Sinusitis may occur in virtually any immunodeficiency disease. The disorders most commonly associated with sinusitis are reviewed in the previous sections. Other immunodeficiency diseases will usually come to clinical attention because of other prominent clinical characteristics prior to the appearance of sinusitis. For example, sinopulmonary disease is a well-known complication of ataxia telangiectasia but children with this disease will come to clinical attention because of ataxia years before their susceptibility to recurrent sinusitis is recognized.

Patients with transient hypogammaglobulinemia of infancy (THI) have recurrent upper respiratory tract infections and while sinusitis has not been frequently reported in this group in the past, the greater awareness of early childhood sinusitis will likely uncover sinusitis in these children as well. These patients come to clinical attention because of increased respiratory infections between 6 and 12 months of age. IgG levels are low and IgA levels are usually reduced, while IgM levels are typically normal. Patients with THI can make antibody to diphtheria and tetanus toxoid and have normal numbers of B- and T-cells. Their hypogammaglobulinemia usually resolves spontaneously at about 2 years of age, although some THI patients will have persistently low IgA levels until age 5 to 6 years.

IMMUNOLOGICAL LABORATORY EVALUATION

There are a large number of laboratory tests available in hospital and commercial laboratories for the evaluation of immune function. Based on our appreciation of the spectrum of immunodeficiency seen in the sinusitis-prone child, a relatively small number of tests are needed to establish an immunologic diagnosis in the vast majority of these patients. These tests are listed in Table 6.2.

If a patient is classified as sinusitis-prone (i.e., three or more episodes of sinusitis within a year or requires 3 or more months of antibiotic therapy for sinusitis), serum immunoglobulin levels (IgG, IgA, IgM, and IgE) as well as IgG subclasses should be measured. If the patient's history suggests respiratory allergy, appropriate allergy skin tests or radioallergosorbent tests (RAST) should be performed. The combination of these tests will detect approximately 75% of the immunodeficient patients and virtually all the allergic patients. If no immunologic abnormalities are found in the initial studies, a blood sample should be obtained for diphtheria and/or tetanus antibody titers, total hemolytic complement, as well as C4 level and a preim-

TABLE 6.2. *Immunological laboratory studies useful in evaluating sinusitis-prone children*

Serum immunoglobulin quantitation (IgG, IgA, IgM, IgE)
Measurement of IgG-subclass levels in serum
Allergy skin testing or radioallergosorbent tests (RAST)
Diphtheria or tetanus antitoxin titers
Pneumococcal polysaccharide immunization with preimmunization and postimmunization antibody titers
Quantitation of peripheral blood B- and T-lymphocytes

munization pneumococcal antibody level. If patients are over 2 years of age but under 6 years, they may be given the pneumococcal vaccine on the same visit. If patients are over 6 years of age, I recommend waiting for the results of the pneumococcal antibody titers to ensure that they are not immune (i.e., antibody levels greater than 300 ng/ml) before administering the vaccine. This practice will avoid painful Arthus reactions at the site of the pneumococcal polysaccharide vaccine inoculation in immune patients. Postimmunization samples should be drawn 3 to 4 weeks after immunization. Antibodies to pneumococcal polysaccharide types 3, 7, 9, and 14 are generally measured and postimmunization levels should exceed 300 ng/ml or the designated protective level for the laboratory used. If patients are found to have low levels of all immunoglobulin, B- and T-lymphocyte populations should be measured in peripheral blood to discriminate between XLA, which lacks B-lymphocytes, and CVID, in which B-cells are usually present. THI patients, who may also be panhypogammaglobulinemic, should have normal B- and T-lymphocyte populations. These studies will also detect disorders with deficiencies of T-cells or T-cell subpopulations.

THERAPY

The management of recurrent/chronic sinusitis in immunodeficient patients is challenging. Vigorous medical management and surgical intervention often fail if the patient is not simultaneously receiving therapy for their underlying immunodeficiency. As noted previously, most sinusitis-prone immunodeficient patients have a deficiency in the ability to produce immunoglobulins and/or antibodies. For patients with global immunoglobulin and antibody deficiencies, such as common variable immunodeficiency and X-linked agammaglobulinemia, immunoglobulin replacement therapy is unequivocally indicated (20,21). For patients with selective IgG-subclass deficiencies and/or selective antibody deficiency, immunoglobulin replacement therapy may be efficacious as indicated by some uncontrolled clinical studies on small numbers of patients (16,22). Efficacy has not as yet been established by double-blind, placebo-controlled trials. Immunoglobulin replacement is not recommended for patients with selective IgA deficiency who do not have an associated IgG-subclass or antibody deficiency. Patients with transient hypogammaglobulinemia of infancy do not require immunoglobulin replacement since they are not thought to be functionally antibody deficient and their defect will resolve generally by 2 years of age (8,21).

Intravenous immunoglobulin (IVIG) infusion is the treatment of choice for immunoglobulin replacement therapy (reviews in refs. 20 and 21). IVIG infusions are superior to intramuscular immunoglobulin injections because more immunoglobulin may be given per treatment, resulting in higher levels of protective circulating antibodies. As a result, prevention of infection is better with IVIG than with intramuscular immunoglobulin injections. In addition, IVIG administration is less painful than intramuscular immunoglobulin injections, an important factor for the older patient who must receive large quantities of immunoglobulin. IVIG therapy is usually begun at a dose of 400 mg per kg of body weight given at 4-week intervals. For details of the infusion procedure the physician should carefully review the instructions in the product package insert as well as review articles on the subject (20,21). Some patients may require more IVIG than others. Serum IgG levels should be checked prior to infusion for the first 3 months of treatment and then at 3-month intervals. Adequate infection control is usually achieved when the preinfusion IgG level is 500 mg/dl higher than that prior to the initiation of immunoglobulin replacement therapy (23). If infection control is inadequate, the interval between infusions may be decreased to 3 weeks or the dose of IVIG may be increased to 600 mg/kg. Patients who are IgA deficient as well as some patients with CVID have IgE anti-IgA antibodies, which may cause anaphylactic reactions if they receive IVIG preparations containing IgA (24). For these patients, the use of an IVIG preparation free of IgA is recommended. When a trial of IVIG therapy is given to children for treatment of IgG-subclass or selective antibody deficiency, patients should be treated for 6 to 12 months and then therapy should be stopped for at least 3 months to permit reevaluation of the patients' need for continued immunoglobulin replacement therapy. The 3-month period off therapy will permit the infused IVIG to be metabolized and then an accurate measure of the patient's own immunoglobulin levels and response to immunization could be determined. If the defects have spontaneously resolved, immunoglobulin replacement may be discontinued and the patient observed. Immunoglobulin replacement therapy is costly, causes some discomfort for the patient, and is time consuming for the parent and medical personnel. It should not be undertaken without careful consideration.

The medical management of episodes of sinusitis in the immunodeficient patient is the same as for nonimmunodeficient patients. Topical measures such as twice daily nasal irrigation with saline followed by a nasal beclomethasone spray help cleanse the mucous membranes and decrease swelling and inflammation. The choice of antibiotics for treatment of infection is based on our understanding of the bacteriology of sinus infections. Unfortunately, little information is available specifically dealing with immunodeficient pa-

tients; however, our preliminary study (11) revealed that cultures taken from the sinuses of immunodeficient patients at surgery were similar to those found by sinus aspiration in nonimmunodeficient children (25–27). *Moraxella catarrhalis, Hemophilus influenzae* (nontypeable), and *Streptococcus pneumoniae* were found, as well as coagulase negative staphylococcus, *Neisseria* species, and anaerobes. In the immunodeficient patients, 90% of the cultures were positive, 50% contained more than one bacterial species, and 30% of the cultures contained anaerobes. These frequencies are all higher than those observed in nonimmunodeficient patients. For antibiotic treatment of acute sinusitis or exacerbations of sinus disease, we generally recommend either amoxicillin with clavulanic acid or erythromycin-sulfisoxazole. Oral cefuroxime axetil has also been found to be helpful, while trimethoprim-sulfa, cefaclor, and cefixime have been less effective in our experience. Patients are treated for 4 weeks and then evaluated clinically and with Waters and Caldwell views of the sinuses. If the patient is clinically well and sinus films are clear, antibiotic therapy may be discontinued and the patient observed. If there is an inadequate response to therapy, the patient should be treated with a different antibiotic and then evaluated after an additional 4 weeks of therapy. At this time, a coronal CT scan of the sinuses is usually performed. If sinus disease persists, the patient should be referred to a pediatric otolaryngologist for consultation.

There is little information published on the surgical management of sinus disease in immunodeficient children. Our own experience is that many immunodeficient patients have undergone some form of sinus surgery without benefit prior to the diagnosis of their immunodeficiency. We recently studied 11 patients with immunodeficiency diseases and chronic sinusitis who underwent endoscopic ethmoidectomy and maxillary antrostomy (11). Four patients had transient immunoglobulin deficiencies while the remaining patients had persistent immune defects. The best outcome was observed in the patients with transient defects. While the patients with persistent defects were symptomatically improved, most continued to require daily antibiotics as well as monthly IVIG therapy. Postoperatively, most of these patients could be maintained symptom free with a single daily dose of prophylactic antibiotic and by rotating antibiotics at 3 to 4 month intervals. Thus, on the basis of preliminary studies, endoscopic ethmoidectomy appears to be very helpful in reestablishing patency of the sinuses once a transient immune defect has resolved. However, further study of the utility of endoscopic surgery in patients with life-long immunodeficiency is required to determine its role in the management of sinus disease in these patients.

REFERENCES

1. Rachelefsky GS, Goldberg M, Katz RM, et al. Sinus disease in children with respiratory allergy. *J Allergy Clin Immunol* 1978;61:310–314.
2. Rachelefsky GS, Shapiro GG. Disease of paranasal sinuses in children. In: Bierman W, Pearlman D, eds. *Management of upper respiratory tract disease*. Philadelphia: Saunders, 1980.
3. Furukawa CT, Rachelefsky GS. Children with sinusitis. *Pediatrics* 1983;71:133–134.
4. Shapiro GG. Sinusitis in children. *J Allergy Clin Immunol* 1988;81:1025–1027.
5. Rachelefsky GS, Katz RM, Siegel SC. Chronic sinusitis in the allergic child. *Pediatr Clin North Am* 1988;35:1091–1101.
6. Rachelefsky GS, Katz RM, Siegel SC. Chronic sinus disease is associated with reactive airways disease in children. *Pediatrics* 1984;73:526–529.
7. Stiehm ER. *Immunologic disorders in infants and children*. Philadelphia: Saunders, 1989.
8. Buckley RH. Immunodeficiency diseases. *JAMA* 1987; 258:2841–2850.
9. Claman HN. The biology of the immune response. *JAMA* 1987;258:2834–2840.
10. Shapiro GG, Virant FS, Furukawa CT, Pierson WE, Bierman CW. Immune defects in patients with refractory sinusitis. *Pediatrics* 1991;89:311.
11. Lusk RP, Polmar SH, Muntz HR. Endoscopic ethmoidectomy and maxillary antrostomy in immunodeficient patients. *Arch Otolaryngol Head Neck Surg* 1991;117:60–63.
12. Shackelford PG, Polmar SH, Mayus JL, Johnson WL, Corry JM, Nahm MN. Spectrum of IgG2 subclass deficiency in children with recurrent infections: prospective study. *J Pediatr* 1986;108:647–653.
13. Soderstrom T, Soderstrom R, Andersson R, Lindberg J, Hanson LA. Factors influencing IgG subclass levels in serum and secretions. *Monogr Allergy* 1988;23:236–243.
14. Oxelius VA, Laurrell AB, Lindquist B, et al. IgG subclasses in selective IgA deficiency. Importance of IgG2–IgA deficiency. *N Engl J Med* 1981;304:1476–1477.
15. Oxelius VA, Berkel AI, Hanson LA. IgG2 deficiency in ataxia-telangiectasia. *N Engl J Med* 1982;306:515–517.
16. Umetsu DT, Ambrosino DM, Quinti I, Silber GR, Geha RS. Recurrent sinopulmonary infections and impaired antibody response to bacterial capsular polysaccharide antigens in children with selective IgG subclass deficiency. *N Engl J Med* 1985;313:1247–1251.
17. Shackelford PG, Granoff DM, Polmar SH, et al. Subnormal serum concentrations of IgG2 in children with frequent infections associated with varied patterns of immunologic dysfunction. *J Pediatr* 1990;116:529–538.
18. Wasserman RL, Barrett D, Burks AW, et al. Antibody deficiency, IgG subclass deficiency and vaccine non-responder states. *Pediatr Infect Dis J* 1990;9:424–433.
19. Rowe PC, McLean RH, Wood RA, Leggiadro RJ, Winkelstein J. Association of homozygous C4B deficiency with bacterial meningitis. *J Infect Dis* 1989;160:448–451.
20. Sorensen RU, Polmar SH. Immunoglobulin replacement therapy. *Ann Clin Res* 1987;19:293–304.
21. Eibl MM, Wedgwood RJ. Intravenous immunoglobulin: a review. *Immunodefic Rev* 1989;1(suppl):1–42.
22. Page R, Friday G, Stillwagon P, Skoner D, Caliguiri L, Fireman P. Asthma and selective immunoglobulin subclass deficiency: improvement of asthma after immunoglobulin replacement therapy. *J Pediatr* 1988;112:127–131.
23. Gelfand EW, Reid B, Roifman CM. Intravenous immune serum globulin replacement in hypogammaglobulinemia. A comparison of high- versus low-dose therapy. *Monogr Allergy* 1988;23:177–186.
24. Burks AW, Sampson HA, Buckley RH. Anaphylactic reactions after gammaglobulin administration in patients with hypogammaglobulinemia. Detection of IgE antibodies to IgA. *N Engl J Med* 1986;314:560–564.
25. Wald ER, Byers C, Guerra N, Casselbrant M, Beste D. Subacute sinusitis in children. *J Pediatr* 1989;115:28–32.
26. Tinkelman DG, Silk HJ. Clinical and bacteriologic features of chronic sinusitis in children. *Am J Dis Child* 1989;143:938–941.
27. Goldenhersh MJ, Rachelefsky GS, Dudley J, et al. The microbiology of chronic sinus disease in children with respiratory allergy. *J Allergy Clin Immunol* 1990;85:1030–1039.

Pediatric Sinusitis,
edited by R. P. Lusk,
Raven Press, Ltd., New York © 1992.

CHAPTER 7

Sinusitis and Asthma

Raymond G. Slavin

The human airway has traditionally been divided into upper and lower segments with clear structural and functional distinctions. Diseases of the upper and lower airways may coexist, with rhinitis and bronchial asthma being good examples. Up to 80% of patients with asthma have rhinitis symptoms while 5 to 15% of patients with perennial rhinitis have asthma. However, little attention has been paid until recently to the possibility that the upper airway may play an important role in the pathogenesis of bronchial asthma. In this chapter, I review the data from both experimental animal and human studies, which indicate that distinctions between upper and lower airways are not as great as previously imagined. There may be important interrelationships with lessons to be learned about the mechanism of disease of one segment of the airway through study of the other segment.

Table 7.1 summarizes the possible relationships between upper and lower airway diseases.

TABLE 7.1. *Association of upper and lower airway disease*

Allergic rhinitis
    Filter function failure; increases allergen/irritant burden on lower airway
    Heat and humidification failure: exercise-induced asthma
    Improvement in pulmonary symptoms by treatment of nasal symptoms
    Increased lower airway responsiveness: specific and nonspecific
Nasal polyps and asthma
Viral upper respiratory tract infection
Nasal–sinus–bronchial reflex

R. G. Slavin: Department of Internal Medicine and Microbiology, Division of Allergy/Immunology, St. Louis University School of Medicine, St. Louis, Missouri 63104-1028.

FILTER FUNCTION FAILURE OF THE NOSE

The nose serves as an important filter of inspired air since all inhaled particles and gases pass through the nose. Relatively large particles are captured by the hairs within the nostrils while other noxious substances are trapped in the mucous (1). It is obvious that nasal obstruction or a failure in the filter function would increase the allergen/irritant burden to the lower airway, thus potentiating lower airway hyperresponsiveness.

HEAT AND HUMIDIFICATION FAILURE

The heating and humidification of inspired air are important functions of the nose. These functions are largely provided by the highly vascularized mucosa of the turbinates and septum. If inspired air bypasses the warming and humidification provided by the nose, then cooler, dryer air is delivered to the lung. This will potentiate the phenomenon referred to as exercise-induced asthma (EIA). Exercise is an important trigger for bronchial asthma and is thought to be initiated by loss of water and heat from the lower airway. Patients can reduce the severity of EIA by breathing through their noses rather than through their mouths during exercise (2).

IMPROVEMENT IN PULMONARY SYMPTOMS BY TREATMENT OF NASAL SYMPTOMS

In a study comparing the efficacy of beclomethasone nasal solution, flunisolide, and cromolyn in relieving symptoms in 120 patients with ragweed allergy, it was noted that 58 patients in this group also had asthma. Surprisingly, all the intranasal treatments considerably reduced the symptoms of seasonal asthma. The authors speculate that intranasally administered drugs restore normal nasal physiologic conditions including warming, humidification, and filtration of airborne allergens (3). It has been shown that a large proportion of ragweed allergen is contained in particles small enough to penetrate the bronchi. These aeroallergens are more likely to deposit in the airways during mouth breathing than during nasal breathing (4).

INCREASED LOWER AIRWAY RESPONSIVENESS IN NASAL DISEASES

Specific

Lower airway sensitivity may be increased in patients who only have clinical evidence of allergic rhinitis. In bronchial challenge studies performed with ragweed allergen, there was considerable overlap in lower airway sensitivity when patients with ragweed asthma were contrasted with patients who have allergic rhinitis. In other words, antigen challenge cannot be used to distinguish patients with hay fever only from those with asthma (5).

Nonspecific

Methacholine, a parasympathomimetic drug, is frequently used in the diagnosis of asthma when spirometry is normal. Asthmatics show an increased bronchoconstrictor response to inhalation of this agent. Twenty-five patients with rhinitis with no evidence of asthma were challenged with methacholine. Ten of these patients showed an increased methacholine response. In five patients, there was also bronchoconstriction in response to hyperventilation and an additional two patients demonstrated increased variability of peak flow rates. Thus, in 7 of 10 patients, increased bronchial responsiveness was confirmed by the use of two different methods, although the patients were asymptomatic. The results indicate that methacholine responsiveness in the asthmatic range is seen in a significant number of patients with rhinitis alone, and that it is associated with variable air flow obstruction and subclinical asthma (6).

Nasal Polyps and Asthma

In a study by Settipane and Chaffee (7) in 1977, 5000 patients with asthma or allergic rhinitis were analyzed. Of the asthma group, 16.7% had polyps and of the 211 total patients with nasal polyps, 70% had asthma. It is estimated that patients with polyps have a 25 to 30% chance of developing bronchial asthma and vice versa (8). Experiments by Kaliner et al. (9) demonstrated that polyps from patients with allergic rhinitis will, on proper stimulation with appropriate antigen, release histamine, leukotrienes, and eosinophil chemotactic factor of anaphylaxis. Interestingly, when polyps from patients with chronic sinusitis are passively sensitized with IgE and then challenged with antigen, there is a greater release of the leukotrienes than histamine. Several studies have offered conflicting evidence of the prevalence of bronchial hyperreactivity in patients with nasal polyps and no history of asthma. One group (10) demonstrated a low response in such subjects to methacholine challenge, while the other showed the opposite effect; that is, bronchial hyperreactivity seemed to be high in these patients, especially in non-atopics (11).

The association of nasal polyps, bronchial asthma, and aspirin sensitivity has been well described. These patients begin with vasomotor rhinitis and profuse rhinorrhea. This is associated later with intense nasal congestion and the development of nasal polyps. Following this, bronchial asthma develops and then, finally, aspirin sensitivity.

INCREASED LOWER AIRWAY REACTIVITY DURING UPPER RESPIRATORY INFECTIONS

Upper respiratory tract infections (URIs) provoke wheezing in many patients who have asthma, both children and adults. It has been only recently appreciated that respiratory viruses most commonly trigger these attacks. Respiratory syncytial virus is most common in young children with rhinovirus and influenza virus being more prevalent in older children and adults (12). The obstructive changes in small airway function of the lung associated with viral illness may persist for up to 5 weeks after the clinical illness has resolved. Viral URIs also cause airway hyperreactivity. The bronchial response to both a specific antigen challenge and a nonspecific challenge with methacholine or histamine are enhanced during a viral URI (13).

A number of mechanisms may explain how viral URIs contribute to airway reactivity, wheezing, and the pathogenesis of asthma.

1. Exfoliation of bronchial epithelium. A viral URI inflames the bronchial epithelium. This will sensitize rapidly adapting sensory vagus fibers located primarily in the epithelium of the large airways. Exposure of these sensitized fibers to an irritant such as histamine causes reflex bronchospasm.
2. Increased permeability of mucous membranes. The inflammation of the bronchial epithelium will allow for increased permeability of antigen.
3. Effect on β-adrenergic function. It is well known that there is a diminished β-adrenergic responsiveness in asthmatics. This basic adrenergic block is enhanced with a viral URI.

TABLE 7.2. *Evidence of nasobronchial reflex*

Investigator	Year	Species	Stimulus	Intervention
Kratchmer	1870	Cat	Ether, SO_2	
Dixon	1903	Cat	Electrical	Sever vagus
Ogura	1964	Humans	Anatomical	Surgery
Speizer	1966	Humans	SO_2	
Kaufman	1969	Humans	Silica	Atropine

4. Augmentation of mediator release. It has been demonstrated that leukocytes of asthmatic patients release increased amounts of histamine when they are incubated with respiratory viruses. This enhanced basophil mediator release appears to be associated with the production of interferon by the viruses.

5. Stimulates synthesis of antiviral IgE. Some respiratory viruses, in particular respiratory syncytial virus and parainfluenza, stimulate the production of allergic antibody IgE to virus (14). The IgE attaches to exfoliated respiratory cells and reacts with the virus to increase the release of histamine, which causes wheezing. Enhanced histamine release causes the virus to produce interferon, which in turn enhances the release of histamine.

NASAL–SINUS–BRONCHIAL REFLEX

A large number of studies have been done over the years relating the nose and paranasal sinuses to asthma (Table 7.2). Most of these studies are predicated on the fact that there are receptors in the nose, the nasopharynx, and presumably the sinuses that, on proper stimulation, result in bronchoconstriction. As long ago as 1870, Kratchmer (15), a French physiologist, could demonstrate a substantial increase in lower airway resistance by stimulating the nose in cats with either ether or sulfur dioxide. In 1903, Dixon and Brodie (16) showed that electrical stimulation of the nose can also result in increased lower airway resistance in cats. They subsequently extended these observations to demonstrate that section of the vagus nerve blocked the changes in lower airway resistance (16).

Ogura and Harvey (17), in looking for an association between nasal resistance and bronchial asthma, conducted a series of experiments in both animal and human subjects. They were able to restore the lower airway to normal in some patients simply by correcting a nasal septal deviation. Speizer and Frank (18) exposed healthy human volunteers to sulfur dioxide intranasally and showed an increase in lower airway reactivity.

In a well controlled study, Kaufman and Wright (19) obtained uniform increases in lower airway resistance by blowing silica particles into the nasopharynx in 10 nonsmoking adults who had no chest complaints and normal pulmonary function tests. Repeating the experiments after the injection of atropine, they demonstrated that the lower airway response was totally obviated.

Could allergy-inducing particles deposited in the nose give rise to a bronchial reflex? No such connection was found in some experimental studies (Table 7.3). When patients with grass- or ragweed-induced allergic rhinitis were subjected to intranasal challenge with specific allergens, no effect on lower airway performance could be demonstrated (20). Schumacher and associates (21), using histamine for intranasal challenge in patients with allergic rhinitis, were similarly unable to show any effect on lower airway responsiveness.

Yan and Salome (22) performed similar studies on patients with perennial rhinitis. When challenged intranasally with histamine, these patients showed a significant fall in forced expiratory volume in 1 s (FEV_1). This would suggest that a certain critical threshold of nasal disease severity may be necessary to provoke reflex changes in the lower airway as a response to nasal challenge (Table 7.4).

TABLE 7.3. *Evidence against nasobronchial reflex*

Investigator	Year	Stimulus	Lower airway
Schumacher	1986	Grass or histamine	No effect
Rosenberg	1983	Ragweed	No effect
Hoehne	1981	Ragweed	No effect

TABLE 7.4. *Response of lower airways to nasal stimulation in asthmatics with rhinitis*

Twelve subjects with perennial allergic rhinitis and stable asthma received a nasal challenge with histamine diphosphate:
  Twelve subjects had greater than sixfold increase in nasal resistance
  Six subjects had greater than 20% fall in FEV_1
  Two subjects had 10 to 17% fall in FEV_1
The airways of some asthmatics narrow in response to nasal stimulation

Data from ref. 22.

RELATIONSHIP OF SINUSITIS AND ASTHMA

The frequent association of paranasal sinus disease and bronchial asthma has been noted for a great many years, but a resurgence of interest in the association became evident only during the past decade. A high incidence of radiographic evidence of sinusitis, on the order of 40 to 60%, has been demonstrated in asthmatic patients in several studies (23,24). The overriding question is, does this association represent an epiphenomenon; that is, are sinusitis and asthma manifestations of the same underlying disease process in different parts of the respiratory tract, or is there a causal relationship, for example, can sinusitis trigger bronchial asthma (25)?

That an association exists between sinus disease and obstructive lung disease has been established, and obviously more objective evidence that sinusitis triggers or exacerbates asthmatic systems is needed. Nevertheless, there are data that indicate that patients who present with difficult to control asthma will improve when coexistent sinusitis is cleared up by medical and/or surgical treatment. This can be considered as strong suggestive evidence for an etiologic role of sinusitis in lower airway disease.

Evidence that sinusitis may have an important etiologic role in asthma may be obtained by examining the effects of adequate medical or surgical treatment of sinusitis on asthmatic manifestations.

Studies by Rachelefsky and associates (26) have demonstrated that children with combined sinusitis and lower airway hyperreactivity show significant improvement of the asthmatic state when they receive appropriate medical treatment for their sinusitis. In Table 7.5, we see the disease characteristics before and after treatment for sinusitis in 48 children with hyperreactive airway disease. Only seven of these children needed sinus lavage. The rest received appropriate medical therapy. As can be seen from the table, 79% of these children were able to discontinue bronchodilators with resolution of their sinusitis. Pulmonary function tests showed normal results in 67% of those with pretreatment abnormalities. It should be emphasized that medical treatment including appropriate antibiotics and decongestants (oral or topical) will generally prove adequate in children with coexistent sinusitis and asthma and surgical intervention is only

TABLE 7.6. *Characteristics of adult patients with combined sinus disease and bronchial asthma*

Asthma preceded by sinusitis (based on history)	>90%
Presence of atopy (based on history and skin tests)	<40%
Aspirin sensitivity (based on history)	>50%
Corticosteroid requirement	>90%

rarely necessary in these cases. Similar results were reported in another group of children with asthma and sinusitis from the University of Pittsburgh (27).

At the St. Louis University Medical Center, we have had an opportunity to observe a large group of adult patients who had coexistent sinusitis and asthma, and who also presented suggestive evidence that the sinusitis played an important role in the pathogenesis of asthma. The characteristics of this group of patients are shown in Table 7.6. More than 90% gave a history indicating that their sinusitis preceded the development of asthma symptoms. Based on history and a battery of allergy skin tests to common St. Louis aeroallergens, two-thirds of the patients were judged to be nonatopic and more than 50% had a history of aspirin sensitivity. Most importantly, more than 90% of these patients were receiving corticosteroids. Corticosteroid dependency furnishes an important clue to those patients in whom an underlying sinus disease may act as a trigger for the development of asthma. These patients were uniformly medically resistant; that is, sinusitis either reoccurred or never sufficiently cleared on aggressive medical management (28).

Our early results obtained with bilateral intranasal sphenoethmoidectomy revealed that 65% of our patients showed significant improvement in their asthmatic state (28). We have found that patients who showed improvement within the 2 years following surgery were likely to have experienced continued improvement throughout a 5-year observation period. More than 80% of the patients reported that they had experienced moderately or greatly improved nasal symptomatology and 60% felt that asthma symptoms had improved. Pretreatment pulmonary function test results improved an average of 20% (29).

TABLE 7.5. *Disease characteristics before and after treatment for sinusitis in 48 children*

Characteristic	Before	After
Cough	100%	29%
Wheeze	100%	15%
Normal PFT	0%	67%
Bronchodilator treatment	100%	21%

Data from ref. 26.

TABLE 7.7. *Tissue eosinophilia in 26 patients with chronic sinusitis*

Group 1	Chronic sinusitis and bronchial asthma (5) marked in all
Group 2	Chronic sinusitis, bronchial asthma, and allergic rhinitis (8) marked in all
Group 3	Chronic sinusitis and allergic rhinitis (7) marked in six
Group 4	Chronic sinusitis marked in none

Data from ref. 31.

POSSIBLE MECHANISMS EXPLAINING THE RELATIONSHIP BETWEEN SINUSITIS AND ASTHMA

Vagal Reflex

The postulated neuroanatomic pathways that could reflexly connect the paranasal sinuses to the lungs are shown in Fig. 7.1. Receptors in the nose, and presumably in the paranasal sinuses, give rise to afferent fibers that in turn form part of the trigeminal nerve. The trigeminal nerve passes to the brain stem, where it can connect via the reticular formation with the dorsal vagal nucleus. From the vagal nucleus, parasympathetic efferent fibers travel in the vagus nerve to the bronchi. The cholinergic (parasympathetic) nervous system plays an integral part in maintaining resting bronchial muscle tone as well as in mediating acute bronchospastic responses. The vagus nerve provides the cholinergic motor supply to airway smooth muscle (30).

The Eosinophil

Evidence suggests that the eosinophil plays an important role in mediating injury to bronchial epithelium in chronic asthma. In a recent study, the role of the eosinophil in chronic inflammatory disease of the paranasal sinuses was investigated with tissue from patients who underwent surgery for chronic sinusitis. As seen in Table 7.7, sinus tissue from patients with sinusitis who also had chronic asthma and/or allergic rhinitis was extensively infiltrated with eosinophils. In contrast, sinus tissue from patients with chronic sinusitis alone had no eosinophils.

Immunofluorescent studies demonstrated a striking association between the presence of extracellular deposition of major basic protein and damage to sinus mucosa. In addition, the histopathology of the paranasal respiratory epithelium appeared similar to that described in bronchial asthma. The findings suggest that the eosinophil acts as an effector cell in chronic inflammatory disease in paranasal respiratory epithelium. This points to the fact that the sinus disease in patients with asthma may be due to the same mechanisms that cause damage to bronchial epithelium (31).

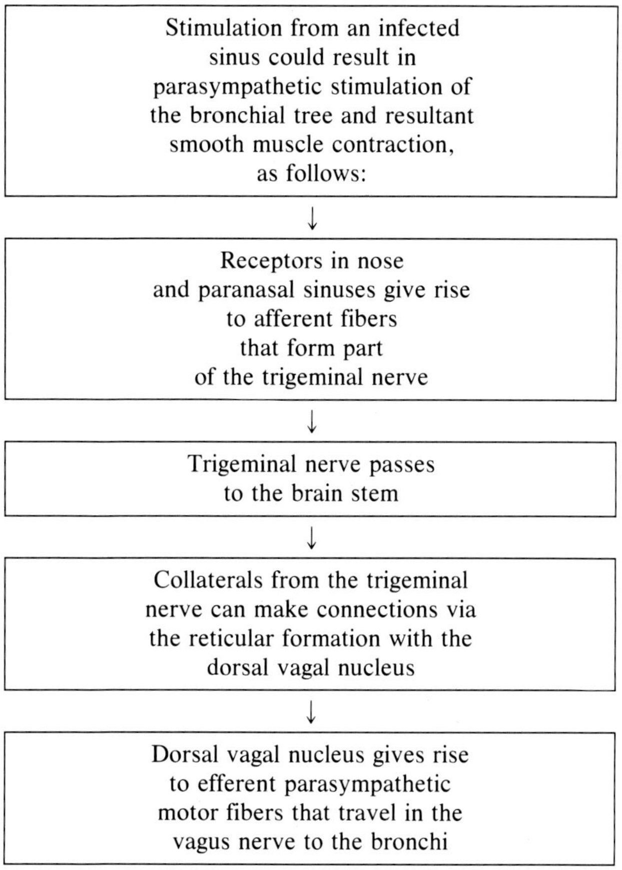

FIG. 7.1. The postulated neural pathways involved in sinusitis-induced bronchospasm.

Inflammatory Mediators

Another proposed mechanism for sinusitis as an aggravator of asthma is local stimulation of irritant receptors with reflex bronchospasm and aspiration of mediators of inflammation into the lower airways. In a recent study, the levels of the leukotrienes, prostaglandin D2, and histamine were measured in maxillary sinus lavage fluid obtained during surgery for chronic sinusitis. These results were compared to levels of mediators in nasal lavage fluid from a group of atopic subjects. The results indicated that the levels of leukotrienes, histamine, and PGD2 were significantly elevated over the control lavage fluid and were in the range associated with local inflammation and irritant receptor stimulation (32) (Table 7.8).

Another recent study from Germany would indicate that aspiration of fluid from the paranasal sinuses does not take place into the lower airway (33).

SUMMARY

It would appear that sinusitis is an important underlying factor for some cases of chronic asthma.

TABLE 7.8. *Inflammatory mediators in lavage fluid*

Procedure	LTC4/D4/E4	Histamine	PGD2
Sinus lavage in chronic sinusitis	1110	258	84
Nasal lavage in atopics	73	6	12

Data from ref. 32.

There is suggestive evidence that sinusitis not only occurs in association with bronchial asthma but may also play a role in its pathogenesis. The basic mechanisms underlying the relationship of sinusitis and asthma need to be investigated and neurophysiologic studies exploring the nature of sinus reflexes should be designed using experimental animal models. There are certainly highly suggestive data to indicate that proper treatment of sinusitis by medical and/or surgical means will frequently result in significant improvement of asthma symptomatology.

REFERENCES

1. Ricketti AJ. Allergic rhinitis. In: Patterson R, ed. *Allergic diseases: diagnosis and management*, 3rd ed. Philadelphia: Lippincott, 1985;207–231.
2. Shturman-Ellstein R, Zeballos RJ, Buckley JM, Souhrado JF. The beneficial effect of nasal breathing on exercise induced bronchoconstriction. *Am Rev Respir Dis* 1978;118:72–76.
3. Welsh PW, Stricker WE, Chi CP, Naessen JM, Reese ME, Reed CE, Marcoux JP. The efficacy of beclomethasone nasal solution, flunisolide, and cromolyn in relieving symptoms of ragweed allergy. *Mayo Clin Proc* 1987;62:125–134.
4. Agarwal MK, Swanson MC, Reed CE, Yuninger JW. Airborne ragweed allergens; association with various particle sizes and short ragweed plant parts. *J Allergy Clin Immunol* 1984;74:687–693.
5. Permutt SM. Bronchial challenge in ragweed sensitive patients. In: Austen KF, Lichtenstein LM, eds. *Asthma: physiology, immunopharmacology and treatment*. Orlando: Academic Press, 1977;chap 17.
6. Ramsdale EH, Morris MM, Roberts RS, Hargreave FE. Asymptomatic bronchial responsiveness in rhinitis. *J Allergy Clin Immunol* 1985;75:573–577.
7. Settipane GA, Chaffee FH. Nasal polyps in asthma and rhinitis: a review of 6,037 patients. *J Allergy Clin Immunol* 1977;59:17–23.
8. Maloney J, Collins J. Nasal polyps and bronchial asthma. *Br J Dis Chest* 1977;41:1–5.
9. Kaliner M, Wasserman SI, Austen KF. Immunologic release of chemical mediators from human nasal polyps. *N Engl J Med* 1973;289:277–282.
10. Downing E. Bronchial reactivity in patients with nasal polyps before and after polypectomy. *J Allergy Clin Immunol* 1983;69:102 (abstract).
11. Miles LR. Methacholine sensitivity in nasal polyposis and effects of polypectomy. *J Allergy Clin Immunol* 1982;69:102 (abstract).
12. Busse WE. The precipitation of asthma by upper respiratory infections. *Chest* 1985:87(suppl);44–48.
13. Eggleston PA, Fish JE. Upper airway disease and bronchial hyperreactivity. *Clin Rev Allergy* 1984;2:429–441.
14. Welliver RC. Upper respiratory infection in asthma. *J Allergy Clin Immunol* 1983;72:341–346.
15. Kratchmer I. Physiologic relationships between nasal breathing and pulmonary function. *Laryngoscopy* 1966;76:30–35.
16. Dixon WE, Brodie TG. The bronchial muscles, their innervation, and the action of drugs upon them. *J Physiol (Lond)* 1903;29:93–97.
17. Ogura JH, Harvey JE. Nasopulmonary mechanisms. Experimental evidence of the influence of the upper airway upon the lower. *Acta Otolaryngol* 1971;71:123–132.
18. Speizer FE, Frank NR. A comparison of changes in pulmonary flow resistance in health volunteers actively exposed to SO_2 by mouth and nose. *Br J Ind Med* 1966;23:75–79.
19. Kaufman J, Wright GW. The effect of nasal and nasopharyngeal irritation on airway resistance in man. *Am Rev Respir Dis* 1969;100:626–630.
20. Hoehne JH, Reed CE. Where is the allergic reaction in ragweed asthma? *J Allergy Clin Immunol* 1971;48:36–39.
21. Schumacher MJ, Cota BS, Taussig LD. Pulmonary response to nasal challenge testing of atopic subjects with stable asthma. *J Allergy Clin Immunol* 1986;78:30–35.
22. Yan K, Salome C. The response of the airways to nasal stimulation in asthmatics with rhinitis. *Eur J Respir Dis* 1983;128(suppl):105–109.
23. Katz R. Sinusitis in children with respiratory allergy. *J Allergy Clin Immunol* 1978;61:190–195.
24. Berman S. Maxillary sinusitis and bronchial asthma: correlation of roentgenograms, cultures and thermograms. *J Allergy Clin Immunol* 1974;53:311–318.
25. Slavin RG. Relationship of nasal disease and sinusitis to bronchial asthma. *Ann Allergy* 1982;49:76–80.
26. Rachelefsky GS, Katz RM, Siegel SC. Chronic sinus disease with associated reactive airway disease in children. *Pediatrics* 1984;783:526–529.
27. Friedman R, Ackerman M, Wald E. Asthma and bacterial sinusitis in children. *J Allergy Clin Immunol* 1984;74:185–189.
28. Slavin RG, Cannon RE, Friedman WH. Sinusitis and bronchial asthma. *J Allergy Clin Immunol* 1980;66:250–257.
29. Mings R, Friedman WH, Linford P, Slavin RG. Five year follow-up of the effects of bilateral intranasal sphenoethmoidectomy in patients with sinusitis and asthma. *Am J Rhinol* 1988;71:123–132.
30. Casale T. Neuromechanisms of asthma. *Ann Allergy* 1987;59:391–399.
31. Harlin SL, Ansel DG, Lane SR, Myers J, Kephart GM, Gleich GJ. A clinical and pathologic study of chronic sinusitis: the role of the eosinophil. *J Allergy Clin Immunol* 1988;81:867–875.
32. Stone BD, Georgitis JW, Matthews B. Inflammatory mediators in sinus lavage fluid. *J Allergy Clin Immunol* 1990;85:22(abstract).
33. Bardin PG, Van Heerden BB, Joubert JR. Absence of pulmonary aspiration of sinus contents in patients with asthma and sinusitis. *J Allergy Clin Immunol* 1990;85:82–88.

Pediatric Sinusitis,
edited by R. P. Lusk,
Raven Press, Ltd., New York © 1992.

CHAPTER 8

Sinusitis and Cystic Fibrosis

David S. Parsons

Cystic fibrosis (CF) is a diffuse systemic disease with many manifestations in the head and neck. Patients with CF frequently suffer from chronic nasal obstruction, nasal polyposis, or sinusitis. In a busy tertiary care otolaryngology practice associated with an active CF clinic, up to 10% of children with chronic sinusitis may be CF patients.

Cystic fibrosis is a genetically transmitted autosomal recessive disease characterized by widespread involvement of the exocrine glands. Approximately 5% of the Caucasian population are carriers of the recessive gene, and 1 in 2000 infants is affected. Multiple organ systems are involved: lungs, gastrointestinal tract, sweat glands, and testes (1). It is the most common life-threatening genetic trait in the Caucasian population and is the major cause of severe chronic lung disease in children (2).

Although we have known about this disorder for more than half a century, our awareness of its head and neck manifestations only became apparent within the past three decades. In 1936, Fanconi et al. (3) recognized the collection of symptoms that subsequently became known as cystic fibrosis. In 1938, Anderson (4) first described this disorder as a clinical entity. But it wasn't until 1959 that Lurie (5) noted the association of cystic fibrosis and nasal polyps. Early in the 1960s, Schwachman et al. (6) published a paper recognizing the relationship between CF and sinusitis.

The majority of articles concerning CF in the head and neck pertain to sinusitis. Our knowledge and awareness of pediatric sinusitis are rapidly expanding, but it remains appropriate to review the existing CF literature.

NONSINUS MANIFESTATIONS OF CYSTIC FIBROSIS OF THE HEAD AND NECK

The salivary glands in children with CF are variably involved. The mucus producing glands have grossly increased ectasia and fibrosis, but sialograms are reported to be normal. The parotid glands, which are primarily serous, have the normal histologic appearance at autopsy (7).

The tracheobronchial tree is frequently abnormal in patients with CF. Chondromalacia has been well described (8). The mucosa may be involved systemically or focally. As in the paranasal sinuses, the secretions become thick and tenacious and cripple ciliary function. Casts of organized secretions have been removed from the lower airway of many children with CF. More than 95% of patients with CF suffer from respiratory tract involvement of varying degrees of severity (9).

The tonsils or adenoids appear to have no involvement in CF (10). Vocal cord paralysis has been reported as the only anomaly of the larynx, and, in each case, this appears to be related to the right heart hypertrophy with compression on the recurrent laryngeal nerve (11).

Jaffe et al. (12) reported that otitis media in cystic fibrosis patients is "remarkably uncommon." Seven studies have shown very limited involvement of the middle ear in these children (10,12–17). Ninety-nine percent of the children in one study had normal or enlarged mastoid air cells (10). Hearing is generally as good as in non-CF children (17). However, children with CF who do develop recurrent otitis media seem to fare less well than normal children and tend to have an increased incidence of cholesteatomas, tympanoplasties, and mastoidectomies (7).

Six studies show the same incidence of allergic disorders in CF patients as in normal children (18–23).

D. S. Parsons: Department of Otolaryngology, Wilford Hall Medical Center, Lackland Air Force Base, Texas 78236.

Surgeons need to be aware that these patients have an increased incidence of bleeding diatheses secondary to the malabsorption of fat-soluble vitamins (12,13). For this reason, prior to surgery, we perform a thorough hematologic workup, which includes an extensive history for bleeding disorders or easy bruisability, CBC with platelets, PT/PTT, and an Ivy bleeding time (24). If the surgical procedure is elective, an autodonor for intraoperative transfusions can be considered.

Paster (25) feels that milder forms of CF exist and may be a partial expression of the disorder. Not all patients exhibit the characteristic picture of GI abnormalities or subsequent failure to thrive. We are currently following two young women with chronic upper and lower respiratory problems, who are both slightly overweight, exhibit no GI symptoms, and have sweat chloride tests repeatedly above 115. An overweight child with recurrent or moderate pulmonary disease will frequently not have CF included in the differential diagnosis. A sweat chloride test should be considered in children with chronic sinus disease as part of the initial workup.

PARANASAL SINUS DISEASE AND CYSTIC FIBROSIS

The major manifestations of CF in the head and neck are the formation of nasal polyps and the development of chronic sinusitis (13,22) (Fig. 8.1).

The reported incidence of nasal polyps in patients with CF is highly variable and ranges from 6 to 48% (7,8,10,12,13,15–19,22,23,26,27). Most papers do not report how the polyps were seen. It is likely that most of the polyps were visualized by non-otolaryngologists using anterior rhinoscopy. The methods available for vasoconstriction and visualization may well have been

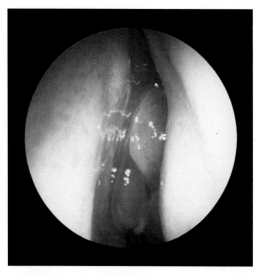

FIG. 8.1. Nasal polyps obstructing the osteomeatal complex and right middle meatus.

substandard. The majority of the papers are retrospective chart reviews and included no reports of the use of microscopes or telescopes. Of greater concern is the failure to document the absence of nasal polyps in CF patients.

Cuyler and Monaghan (19), reporting on CF patients who had been referred to an otolaryngologist for chronic sinusitis symptoms, noted that 100% of the patients had nasal polyps. While recognizing that this is a skewed population, it remains unclear whether nasal polyps exist in CF patients without the presence of sinusitis.

Several authors reported the peak incidence of the presence of nasal polyps to be between ages 5 and 14 years (12,13,16,19,26). No reason is offered why, after age 14, the polyps would become less common. We do know that when many of these papers were published, children with CF frequently did not survive adolescence. Of those who did survive, it was not determined whether they had less severe disease or a variable expression of the disease, or offered fewer complaints of symptoms because they had learned to "live with their disease."

No paper has yet described a CF child less than 2 years old with nasal polyposis. Quite possibly, this may be secondary to poor nasal examinations in this age group or the failure of small polyps to produce significant symptoms. Nasal polyps have been identified by the author in non-CF children with unremitting chronic sinusitis who were less than age 2 at the time of sinus surgery.

Kulczycki et al. (9) reported in 1970 that the nasal mucosa in CF patients becomes hyperplastic with prominent turbinates, which occasionally conceal the nasal polyps. Children with chronic nasal symptoms often manifest edematous mucosa, and the anterior portion of the inferior turbinate may be swollen against the septum, making visualization of the remainder of the nose extremely difficult. With a presentation such as this, the absence of nasal polyps cannot be determined by anterior rhinoscopy alone. Narrowing of the nasal passages and ostia of the paranasal sinuses secondary to mucosal hypertrophy may prevent adequate sinus drainage.

The data regarding the natural history of polyps in CF are incomplete. As previously mentioned, several studies report that the polyps actually decrease after age 14 (12,13,19). It is interesting to note, however, that the highest incidence of nasal polyps, 48%, was reported in adults (22). No studies report prospective evaluations using vasoconstrictors and telescopes. It is likely that the incidence of nasal polyposis in children with CF is much higher than previously reported. As patients with this disorder live longer, we will be able to obtain a better assessment of the natural history of polypoid disease in cystic fibrosis.

The occurrence of radiographic abnormalities of the paranasal sinuses in children with CF is quite striking (28). Eight papers reviewed indicated that 100% of all CF patients had positive plain sinus x-rays (10,13,16,18,21,22,24,26), and an additional four papers noted abnormalities in 90 to 96% (6,19,29,30). The likelihood of a positive sinus series in a child with CF will approximate 98%. Since it can therefore be stated with some assurance that virtually all children with CF will have a positive sinus series, there probably is little value in repeating plain sinus films once the diagnosis of CF has been verified. All subsequent sinus series will most likely be positive, and the only benefit for repeat plain sinus series would be to follow an existing air–fluid level. Medical therapy will not cure the sinus disease and subsequent x-rays will be of very limited help with therapeutic decisions. As a result, CF patients should be followed clinically rather than radiographically.

The primary medical provider, or the surgeon, must ask whether sinus series are justified. The accuracy of these x-rays has already been determined to be poor, based on a recent study (31), and the appropriateness of sinus series in follow-up is highly questionable.

Information regarding computerized tomography of the paranasal sinuses in CF is quite limited. The only published study to date (19) involves children referred to an otolaryngologist for evaluation of sinusitis; these children all had positive CT scans. Our experience is identical, but neither group gives a fair representation of all patients with CF. Diamant et al. (32) suggests that 50% of *all* children having CT scans will demonstrate positive findings within the paranasal sinuses.

The coronal CT scan has become the "gold standard" of radiographic studies for determining the extent of disease in the paranasal sinuses. Magnetic resonance imaging (MRI) is more expensive and requires at least the same, if not a deeper, level of sedation in a smaller child. There is concern that MRI may overcall disease in the paranasal sinuses.

Do children with CF and abnormal radiographs actually have clinical disease? It is apparent that patients with this disorder have a high propensity for developing sinusitis. On careful questioning, if the child is asymptomatic, should an extensive workup be done? Will the patient's or family's awareness of a positive radiograph or CT scan exacerbate clinical symptoms?

In 1971, Neeley et al. (10) stated: "It was amazing to find that our patients had relatively few nasal symptoms until questioned intensively on this point." All studies conducted prior to this to verify the presence of clinical sinusitis in CF patients were retrospective and uniformly found a low incidence of sinusitis, ranging from 4 to 15% (13,16,30). An autopsy study, however, revealed 34% (8,31). The study by Neely and co-

workers was a prospective study and revealed an incidence of 93%. These CF patients had clinical and historical evidence of sinusitis.

The clinical diagnosis of sinusitis is best verified by a thorough history. The physical examination has not been found to be an effective determinant of the presence or absence of active disease in any consistent fashion. In non-CF children, Wald et al. (33) have defined a triad of symptoms obtained from the history which are most frequently found in sinusitis: purulent nasal discharge with obstruction, cough that may persist during the daytime but is typically worse at night or in the early morning, and malodorous breath. At Wilford Hall USAF Medical Center (WHMC), we have identified headaches to be present in more than 90% of non-CF children with chronic sinusitis who were older than 18 months. Additionally, this study found that children tend to have significant behavioral changes with exacerbations of acute sinusitis or in the presence of chronic sinusitis (34). These behavioral changes may be subtle or quite striking and include abnormal psychiatric behavior. The presentations of sinusitis in children with CF are no different. Additional symptoms that are present less frequently include chronic middle ear disorders, sore throats, hoarse voice, fever, dental pain, a bad taste in the mouth, and facial tenderness. Many patients describe acute severe facial pain after bending over and then rising.

Regarding the physical examination, children with CF have a low incidence of otitis media, so the ear evaluation is frequently normal. Bilateral adenopathy is usually present in these children because of the frequency of the upper respiratory illnesses. The remainder of the head and neck examination tends to be normal except for the nose. Often these children will have purulent nasal discharge with swollen nasal mucosa. Seeing beyond the anterior inferior turbinate is often difficult, but if adequate vasoconstriction and a telescope are used, nasal polyposis can often be identified. Transillumination has been recognized to be a poor diagnostic test for children who do not have CF and who present with symptoms compatible with sinusitis (35). Children with CF will more than likely have polypoid thickening in the sinus mucosa, and transillumination will not occur even after medical therapy.

The age of onset of first sinusitis symptoms has been reported to be around the age of 5 in CF children (16,18). However, very little is written regarding the clinical presentation of sinus disease in CF. Neeley et al. (10) stated that children aged 2 to 4 tend to have "stuffy and snuffly noses, but this improves after age four." The parents of CF children at WHMC, when questioned intensely, usually offered that the nasal or sinus symptoms had essentially "always been there." Otolaryngologists are now much more aware that children, including infants and toddlers, can develop sinusitis; small children with CF must be suspected of harboring this disease.

Rulon et al. (36), in 1963, discussed the functional and histological manifestations of CF polyps. They said that the viscous mucus present in these children leads to cystic dilatation of the nasal mucus glands, thereby causing compression and obstruction of the terminal capillaries. Fluid transudation then occurred, which led to the edematous stromal changes and polypoid prolapse.

Studies vary regarding the beat frequency of the cilia (37,38) but histologically the cilia appear to be normal (10). There does exist a decreased beat frequency with slowed mucociliary transport, but this may be due to the increased viscosity of the nasal mucus. The mucus created is 30 to 60 times more viscous in CF than in non-CF patients. The tenacious secretions are so thick that the ciliary function is crippled and the flow of mucus is quite delayed (7).

Nasal polyps have histologic differences that can be identified (7). The polyps are *not* reported to have increased vascularity. Two pathologic studies stated that the vascularity was "normal" and that "vessels were not exceedingly abundant" (10,18).

The primary organism most responsible for sinusitis in CF is *Pseudomonas aeruginosa* (8,16,18,22,30). *Staphylococcus aureus* has been reported to be the second most common pathogen (8,18,22). Shapiro et al. (30) state that *Hemophilus influenzae* is a frequent causative organism. There are no obvious correlations between the cultures of the sinus washouts and the corresponding sputum samples or nasopharyngeal and throat cultures (23,30). If it is essential to know the organism, the only effective method of collection so far described is a sinus tap.

SURGICAL THERAPY FOR SINUS DISEASE IN CF

The presence of clinical sinusitis in CF children may be much higher than has been reported previously in the literature. As we become more aware of this, the inclination may be to identify children with CF as early surgical candidates. However, early surgical intervention should be avoided until a well-defined complex of symptoms indicating the need for surgery exists. Sinus surgery is clearly not curative in CF. At WHMC, we only consider for surgery CF children who have significant symptomatic nasal obstruction, severe paranasal sinus disease unresponsive to medical management, postnasal drip exacerbating the child's pulmonary disease, or poorly controlled pulmonary disease with contributing sinusitis.

Preoperative hospitalization frequently is not required in children with CF (26); however, the pul-

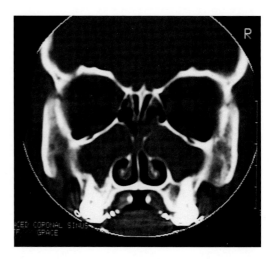

FIG. 8.2. A coronal CT scan demonstrating medial displacement of the middle turbinates and medial wall of the maxillary antrum. The maxillary sinus was found to be filled with polyps and purulence.

monary and nutritional status of these children must be optimized. This often can be performed on an outpatient basis, but preoperative iv antibiotics may be necessary. Many CF families are already aware of the benefits of home iv therapy.

At WHMC, we gave oral prednisone (2 mg/kg/day b.i.d.) 10 to 14 days preoperatively and have found this to be extremely effective in shrinking nasal polyposis and thus improving the surgeon's visualization of the surgical landmarks. Despite what has been reported regarding polyp vascularity, blood loss has been decreased with the shrinkage of the polyps. The surgeon must remember that the most frequent cause of complications in intranasal sinus surgery is poor visibility because of inadequately controlled hemostasis. A rapid tapering off of the steroids can be accomplished postoperatively, assuming a stable pulmonary status.

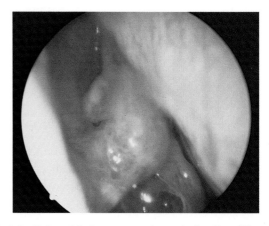

FIG. 8.3. Polypoid changes to the anterior tip of the right middle turbinate with subsequent development of synechiae.

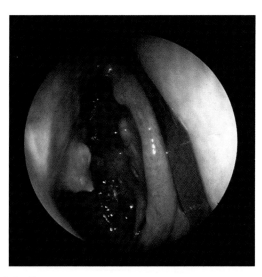

FIG. 8.4. Early postoperative view of the right middle meatus of the patient in Fig. 8.2. The middle turbinate is still strikingly flat and medially displaced.

The preoperative steroids probably do little to prevent postoperative recurrence of the polyps, so topical nasal steroids should be instituted immediately following the procedure. Intraoperative preparations for hemostasis are no different from those for other patients.

Jaffe et al. (12) reported several findings in 1977 which remain characteristic of sinus surgery in CF patients. They noted that the middle turbinate was often pushed flush against the septum (Fig. 8.2) and that polypoid changes existed at the tip of the middle and inferior turbinates (Fig. 8.3). Septal deviation was not uncommon secondary to polyposis. The medial maxillary sinus wall was dilated into the nasal cavity (Fig. 8.2). Often there was destruction of this same wall near the natural ostium so that with removal of the polyps,

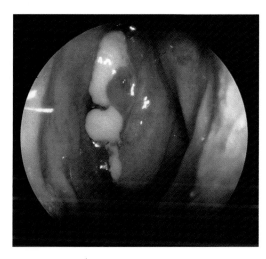

FIG. 8.5. Mucopus in the right middle meatus with polyps. Purulence and polyps were found in all the sinus cavities.

or with shrinkage of the polyps with steroids, an adequate middle meatus antrostomy was already identifiable. One of the most striking features was the enormous number of polyps and the difficulty in localizing the middle turbinate. This structure was typically against the septum with the turbinate pressed thin by the expanding polyps in the middle meatus (Fig. 8.4). Mucopus in the middle meatus was a common finding (Fig. 8.5).

SURGICAL RESULTS

A high incidence of polypoid recurrence following polypectomy alone has been reported (7,13,26); the frequency of clinically significant recurrence has varied between 60 and 87% (12,26). Based on the data reported to date, a polypectomy alone should be regarded as inadequate. However, it is the most common surgical procedure, after laparotomy, that CF children undergo (13).

The extent of intranasal surgery of polyposis was found to be inversely proportional to the recurrence rate (13). The recurrence rate of polyps varied from 13 to 53% if a polypectomy is used in combination with a classic sinus procedure (13,22). The classic sinus procedures include the Caldwell–Luc, intranasal or external ethmoidectomies, and nasal antral windows (NAWs). Neeley et al. (10) reported that there was not enough clinical or radiographic change in a postoperative patient to indicate that the NAWs should be continued in the armamentarium of the sinus surgeon. Muntz and Lusk (39) have shown that NAWs are ineffective surgical therapy in children without CF who suffer with chronic sinusitis.

Functional endoscopic sinus surgery (FESS) is now being used with greater frequency for children with chronic sinusitis. However, in children with CF, no long-term studies with adequate follow-up have been performed. Based on early unreported data from San Antonio, St. Louis, and Edmonton, Canada, patients with CF who have undergone FESS have had significant improvement in their sinus and pulmonary symptomatology. Nasal polyps have recurred in virtually all patients, but most have not been symptomatically obstructive. These children have uniformly been followed with vasoconstrictive agents and telescopes, thus allowing a more thorough postoperative evaluation.

In San Antonio, if a child with CF is sufficiently symptomatic to undergo a major sinus operation, we have found that virtually every sinus is involved; we therefore perform FESS with a total sphenoethmoidectomy opening the natural frontal and maxillary sinus ostia. The need for secondary revision surgery within the first 3 years of follow-up has been approximately 50%; but in all cases, the families felt that the children were significantly improved following the first procedure. The criterion for revision surgery has been the recurrence of offending sinus symptoms, but none of the patients experienced symptoms that were as troublesome as preoperatively.

No determination has been made regarding the advantages of FESS over classic sinus procedures, nor has any substantive data been available to show that a more extensive FESS is better than a limited procedure. However, all patients who underwent sinus surgery in the three institutions had pansinusitis with disease present in each sinus cavity. Most of these patients have only required hospitalization for one postoperative night, because optimal outpatient preoperative and postoperative medical care has been available.

As our knowledge of pediatric sinusitis continues to grow, it is apparent that the information available regarding this disorder in the CF literature is inadequate. Cystic fibrosis in the head and neck, with particular emphasis on the paranasal sinuses, is a rapidly expanding field with tremendous opportunities for clinical research.

REFERENCES

1. Kempe, Silver, O'Brien, Fulginiti. *Current pediatric diagnosis and treatment*, 9th ed. Los Altos, CA: Lange, 1987.
2. Behrman V. *Nelson's textbook of pediatrics*, 13th ed. Philadelphia: Saunders, 1987.
3. Fanconi G, Wehlinger E, Knauer C. Das coeliakie syndrom bei angeborenger zysticher pancreas fibromatose and bronchictasein. *Weiner Med Wochenschr* 1936;86:753–756.
4. Anderson D. Cystic fibrosis of the pancreas and its relation to coeliac disease: a clinical and pathologic study. *Am J Dis Child* 1938;56:344–399.
5. Lurie MH. Cystic fibrosis of the pancreas and the nasal mucosa. *Ann Otol Rhinol Laryngol* 1959;68:478.
6. Schwachman H, Kukychi I, Mueller H, Flake C. Nasal polyps in patients with cystic fibrosis. *Pediatrics* 1962;30:389–401.
7. Kramer RI. Otorhinolaryngolic complications of cystic fibrosis. *Otolaryngol Clin North Am*, 1977;10(1):205–208.
8. Vawter GF, Schwachman H. Cystic fibrosis in adults: an autopsy study. *Pathology Annu*, 1979;14(Pt 2):357–382.
9. Kulczycki LL, Herer GR, Butler JS. Cystic fibrosis and hearing. Integrity of the upper respiratory tract as related to hearing sensitivity. *Clin Pediatr (Phila)* 1970;9(7):138–140.
10. Neely JG, Harrison GM, Jerger JF, Greenberg SD, Presberg H. The otolaryngologic aspects of cystic fibrosis. *Trans Am Acad Ophthalmol Otolaryngol*, 1972;76(2):313–324.
11. Zitsch RP, Reilly JS. Vocal cord paralysis associated with cystic fibrosis. *Ann Otol Rhinol Laryngol* 1987;96(Nov–Dec):680–683.
12. Jaffe BF, Strome M, Khaw KT, Schwachman H. Nasal polypectomy and sinus surgery for cystic fibrosis—a 10 year review. *Otolaryngol Clin North Am* 1977;10(1):81–90.
13. Cepero R, Smith RJ, Catlin FI, Bressler KL, Furata GT, Shandera KC. Cystic fibrosis—an otolaryngologic perspective. *Otolaryngol Head Neck Surg* 1987;97(4):356–360.
14. Todd NM, Martin WS. Temporal bone pneumatization in cystic fibrosis. *J Infect Dis* 1982;146(5):589–593.
15. Taylor B, Evans JN, Hope GA. Upper respiratory tract in cystic fibrosis. Ear–nose–throat surveys of 50 children. *Arch Dis Child* 1974;49(2):133–136.
16. Cunningham DG, Gatti WM, Eitenmiller AM, Van Gorder PN. Cystic fibrosis: involvement of the ear, nose and paranasal sinuses. *IMJ* 1975;470–474.
17. Bak-Pederson K, Larsen PK. Inflammatory middle ear disease in patients with cystic fibrosis. *Acta Otolaryngol [Suppl] (Stockh)* 1979;360:138–140.
18. Magid SL, Smith CC, Dolowitz DA. Nasal respiratory changes in cystic fibrosis of the pancreas. Trans Pacific Coast Oto-Ophthalmological Society Annual Meeting 1966, vol 47, pp 81–89.
19. Cuyler JP, Monaghan AJ. Cystic fibrosis and sinusitis. *J Otolaryngol* 1989;18(4):173–175.
20. Drake-Lee AB, Pitcher-Wilmott RW. The clinical and laboratory correlates of nasal polyps in cystic fibrosis. *Int J Pediatr Otorhinolaryngol* 1982;4(3):209–214.
21. Berman JM, Colman BH. Nasal aspects of cystic fibrosis in children. *J Laryngol Otol* 1977;91(2):133–139.
22. Crockett DM, McGill TJ, Healy GB, Friedman EM, Salkeld LJ. Nasal and paranasal sinus surgery in children with cystic fibrosis. *Ann Otol Rhinol Laryngol* 1987;96(4):367–372.
23. Drake-Lee AB, Morgan DW. Nasal polyps and sinusitis in children with cystic fibrosis. *J Laryngol Otol* 1989;103(8):753–755.
24. Bolger WE, Parsons DS. Preoperative hemostatic assessment of the adenotonsillectomy patient. *Otolaryngol Head Neck Surg* 1990;103:396–405.
25. Paster SB. Nasal polyposis and sinusitis in cystic fibrosis. *Rocky Mt Med J* 1976;73(5):261–263.
26. Reilly JS, Kenna MA, Stool SE, Bluestone CD. Nasal surgery in children with cystic fibrosis: complications and risk management. *Laryngoscope* 1985;95(12):1491–1493.
27. Stern RC, Boat TF, Wood RE, Matthews LW, Doershik CF. Treatment and prognosis of nasal polyps in cystic fibrosis. *Am J Dis Child* 1982;136(12):1067–1070.
28. Ledesma-Medina J, Osman MZ, Gidany BR. Abnormal paranasal sinuses in patients with cystic fibrosis of the pancreas. *Pediatr Radiol* 1989;9:61–64.
29. Gharib R, Allen R, Jous HA. Paranasal sinuses in cystic fibrosis. *Am J Dis Child* 1964;108:499–502.
30. Shapiro ED, Milmoe GJ, Wald ER, Rodnan JB, Bowen AD. Bacteriology of the maxillary sinuses in patients with cystic fibrosis. *J Infect Dis* 1982;146(5):589–593.
31. McAlister WH, Lusk RP, Muntz HR. Comparison of plain radiographs and coronal CT scans in infants and children with recurrent sinusitis. *Am Roentgen Ray Soc* 1989;153(Dec):1259–1264.
32. Diamant MJ, Senac MD, Gilsanz V, Baker S, Gillespie T, Larssen S. Prevalence of incidental paranasal sinuses opacification in pediatric patients: a CT study. *J Comput Assist Tomogr* 1987;11:426–431.
33. Wald ER, Milmoe GJ, Bowen AD, Ledesma-Medina J, Salamon N, Bluestone CD. Acute maxillary sinusitis in children. *N Engl J Med* 1981;304(3):749–754.
34. Parsons DS, Phillips S. FES for treatment of chronic sinusitis in children, presented at SENTAC, Santa Monica CA, 1989 (publication pending).
35. Otten FWA, Grote JJ. The diagnostic value of transillumination for maxillary sinusitis in children. *Int J Pediatr Otorhinolaryngol* 1989;18:9–11.
36. Rulon JT, Brown HA, Logan BG. Nasal polyps and cystic fibrosis of the pancreas. *Arch Otolaryngol* 1963;78:192–199.
37. Rutland H, Cole PJ. Nasal mucociliary clearance and ciliary beat frequency in cystic fibrosis compares with sinusitis and bronchiectasis. *Thorax* 1981;36(9):654–658.
38. Magid SL, Smith CC, Dolowitz DA. Nasal mucosa in pancreatic cystic fibrosis. *Arch Otolaryngol* 1967;86(2):212–216.
39. Muntz HR, Lusk RP. Nasal antral windows in children: a retrospective study. *Laryngoscope* 1990;100(6):643–646.

Pediatric Sinusitis,
edited by R. P. Lusk,
Raven Press, Ltd., New York © 1992.

CHAPTER 9

Medical Management of Sinusitis in Pediatric Patients

Ellen R. Wald

The mainstay of medical therapy for acute sinusitis is the use of antimicrobial agents. The selection of an antimicrobial requires an appreciation of the usual bacterial pathogens responsible for sinus infection. In the case of acute sinusitis, the common bacterial isolates are *Streptococcus pneumoniae*, *Moraxella catarrhalis*, and *Hemophilus influenzae* in a relative prevalence of 30%, 20%, and 20%, respectively (1). Currently, in Pittsburgh, approximately 75% of *M. catarrhalis* and 30% of *H. influenzae* can be assumed to be β-lactamase producing. Accordingly, about 20% of maxillary sinus pathogens will be resistant to amoxicillin.

COMPARISON OF TREATMENT REGIMENS

Table 9.1 shows those antimicrobials that have been compared in the treatment of children with sinusitis in published studies or abstracts. Theoretically, antimicrobials that are effective against β-lactamase producing bacterial species should offer a therapeutic advantage over amoxicillin in treating 20% of the bacterial isolates responsible for sinusitis. However, it is known that patients with acute sinusitis have a spontaneous cure rate of approximately 40% (3). Therefore about half (10%) of the patients harboring β-lactamase producing organisms in their maxillary sinuses will recover even when not receiving an optimal antimicrobial agent. Accordingly, we can expect to see at most about a 10% difference between regimens that are effective and those that are not effective against β-lactamase producing bacterial species. To demonstrate a

10% difference between any two treatments would require the study of many hundreds of patients in each group of a controlled trial. Most studies of antimicrobial efficacy have involved small numbers of patients—usually between 25 and 30 patients. Therefore, not surprisingly, most antimicrobials have appeared to perform similarly in studies evaluating the clinical outcomes of patients with sinusitis.

Unfortunately, there have been no studies performed in children in which bacteriologic efficacy has been assessed by sinus aspiration and culture after treatment has been initiated. However, several such investigations have been conducted in adults with acute maxillary sinusitis. Table 9.2 shows the bacteriologic efficacy of several different antimicrobial regimens. The follow-up sinus aspiration was performed on the tenth day of treatment. A bacteriologic cure was defined as a sterile aspirate or one in which there had been a reduction in the density of infection by a titer of more than 10^4 colony-forming units/milliliter. Although these studies were performed on adults, similar results would be expected in children.

CHOICE OF ANTIMICROBIALS FOR SINUSITIS

Table 9.3 shows a list of suggested antimicrobials and dosage schedules for use in pediatric patients with acute sinusitis. All of them except cefixime have been used in published studies of children with sinusitis.

Amoxicillin is the drug of choice in patients who present with uncomplicated sinusitis. Amoxicillin has largely replaced ampicillin in the treatment of bacterial complications of upper respiratory tract infections. Amoxicillin is twice as well absorbed as ampicillin and has a longer half-life. Accordingly, it can be prescribed

E. R. Wald: Department of Pediatrics, University of Pittsburgh School of Medicine, Children's Hospital of Pittsburgh, Pittsburgh, Pennsylvania 15213.

TABLE 9.1. *Clinical studies of antibiotics for maxillary sinusitis in children*

Reference	Drugs and dosage regimen	Clinical cure Number	Clinical cure Percentage
1	Amoxicillin, 40 mg/kg/day in 3 divided doses	22/27	81
	Cefaclor, 40 mg/kg/day in 3 divided doses	18/23	78
2	Cefaclor, 40 mg/kg/day in 3 divided doses	11/12	92
	Amoxicillin/potassium clavulanate, 40 mg/kg/day in 3 divided doses	16/17	93
3	Amoxicillin, 40 mg/kg/day in 3 divided doses	20/30	67
	Amoxicillin/potassium clavulanate, 40 mg/kg/day in 3 divided doses	18/28	64
4	Amoxicillin, 50 mg/kg/day in 4 divided doses	22/22	100
	Erythromycin/sulfisoxazole, 50/150 mg in 4 divided doses	21/22	95
5	Amoxicillin, 40 mg/kg/day in 3 divided doses	17/22	77
	Erythromycin ethylsuccinate, 30–40 mg/kg/day in 4 divided doses	8/22	36
	Sulfamethoxazole–trimethoprim, 40/8 mg/kg/day in 2 divided doses	13/21	62

in half the dose of ampicillin and three rather than four times daily. Amoxicillin is effective in most patients, relatively inexpensive, and, most importantly, safe. Safety must be a prime consideration when treating a condition that has a spontaneous cure rate of 40%. The only disadvantage of amoxicillin is its susceptibility to the action of the β-lactamases produced by some *H. influenzae* and *M. catarrhalis*. To overcome this problem, Augmentin, an oral agent in which amoxicillin is combined with potassium clavulanate, was developed and marketed beginning in 1985. Potassium clavulanate is the salt of clavulanic acid, a β-lactam with barely any activity against bacterial pathogens but capable of effective inhibition of β-lactamase enzymes. Amoxicillin/potassium clavulanate is equivalent to amoxicillin alone in activity against amoxicillin-susceptible organisms. The addition of clavulanic acid extends the spectrum of amoxicillin to include β-lactamase producing strains of *H. influenzae*, *M. catarrhalis*, *Staphylococcus aureus*, and anaerobic bacteria. Amoxicillin/potassium clavulanate causes gas-

trointestinal symptoms such as abdominal pain, nausea, and diarrhea; however, the diarrhea is often tolerable and, if not, is immediately and predictably reversed when the agent is discontinued.

Erythromycin/sulfisoxazole is a combination oral agent with an appropriate spectrum for the treatment of sinusitis in children. Erythromycin, effective against gram-positive cocci, cannot be used alone in the treatment of acute sinusitis because it provides inadequate coverage for *H. influenzae*, an important etiologic agent in all age groups. Erythromycin/sulfisoxazole is usually recommended to be administered four times daily and has the potential for gastrointestinal discomfort and hypersensitivity to the sulfa component. The latter, although infrequent, is more serious and potentially less easily reversed than toxicity observed with β-lactams.

Sulfamethoxazole–trimethoprim (SMX-TMP) is another alternative option for oral treatment. The combination of these two folic acid antagonists provides a broad spectrum of antimicrobial activity. SMX-TMP

TABLE 9.2. *Studies of bacteriologic cure in adult patients with acute maxillary sinusitis conducted by the Charlottesville (VA) group*

Reference	Drug and dosage regimen	Satisfactory bacteriologic cure for sinusitis confirmed via aspiration and culture Number	Satisfactory bacteriologic cure for sinusitis confirmed via aspiration and culture Percentage
6	Ampicillin, 2.0 g in 4 divided doses	12/13	92
	Amoxicillin, 1.5 g in 3 divided doses	14/14	100
	SMX-TMP, 320/1600 mg in 2 divided doses[a]	18/19	95
	Cefaclor, 1.0 g in 2 divided doses	1/5	20
	Cefaclor, 2.0 g in 4 divided doses	16/17	94
7	Bacampicillin, 1.6 g in 2 divided doses	18/19	95
8	Cyclacillin, 1.5 g in 3 divided doses	23/26	88
	Amoxicillin, 1.5 g in 3 divided doses	25/27	93
9	Cefuroxime axetil, 0.5 g in 2 divided doses	36/38	95
	Cefaclor, 1.5 g in 3 divided doses	15/21	71

Adapted from ref. 9.
[a] SMX-TMP, sulfamethoxazole–trimethoprim.

TABLE 9.3. *Antimicrobials and dosage schedules for the treatment of sinusitis in children*

Antimicrobial	Dosage
Amoxicillin	40 mg/kg/day in 3 divided doses
Amoxicillin/potassium clavulanate	40/10 mg/kg/day in 3 divided doses
Erythromycin/sulfisoxazole	50/150 mg/kg/day in 4 divided doses
Sulfamethoxazole–trimethoprim	40/8 mg/kg/day in 2 divided doses
Cefaclor	40 mg/kg/day in 3 divided doses
Cefuroxime axetil	250 or 500 mg in 2 divided doses
Cefixime	9 mg/kg/day in 1 dose

is inexpensive and is given only twice daily. Once again, sulfa hypersensitivity is a potential problem. Moreover, SMX-TMP does not provide adequate antimicrobial coverage for Group A streptococci. This may be an important coinfecting organism in approximately 20% of patients with acute sinusitis (3). Of interest, *S. pneumoniae* has recently been reported to demonstrate increasing resistance to SMX-TMP in communities where SMX-TMP is frequently used to treat respiratory infections. In a recent prospective study of children in day care, the prevalence of SMX-TMP-resistant *S. pneumoniae* increased from 5% in 1979 to 30% in 1984 (10). The emergence of resistance among *S. pneumoniae* may eventually limit the usefulness of this combination antimicrobial agent.

The cephalosporins are antimicrobials that are structurally similar to the penicillins and are also classified as β-lactam antimicrobials. They have been categorized as first, second, and third generation agents according to their time of introduction and similarity of *in vitro* characteristics. The first generation cephalosporins lack sufficient activity against *H. influenzae* and therefore are not attractive for use in the treatment of otitis media or sinusitis. Cefaclor, a second generation cephalosporin, has been a popular oral drug for the treatment of respiratory infections in children in part because of its pleasant taste. Unfortunately, cefaclor is susceptible to the action of the β-lactamases produced by most strains of *M. catarrhalis* and some strains of *H. influenzae*. When given twice daily for otitis media, the bacteriologic efficacy of cefaclor was only 71% compared to 90% for SMX-TMP (11). A bacteriologic cure was achieved only once when cefaclor, at a dose of 500 mg twice daily, was prescribed for five adults with acute sinusitis (6). These data suggest that when prescribing cefaclor, a three times daily regimen is preferred. Cefaclor has also been associated with a serum sickness-like reaction in children who have received multiple courses of the drug. The incidence of this reaction is approximately 1.0% (12).

In contrast to cefaclor, cefuroxime axetil, another second generation cephalosporin, is a very attractive option for the treatment of older children with sinusitis who require an antimicrobial with a more expanded spectrum than amoxicillin. When cefaclor at 500 mg three times daily was compared to cefuroxime axetil at 250 mg twice daily in the treatment of acute maxillary sinusitis in adults, the bacteriologic cure rates were 71% and 95%, respectively ($p < 0.05$ Fisher's exact test) (9). Cefuroxime is resistant to the action of the β-lactamases produced by *H. influenzae*, *M. catarrhalis*, and *S. aureus*. In its parenteral form, it has enjoyed a great deal of popularity for the treatment of serious infections of the upper and lower respiratory tracts of children. Unfortunately, in oral form, cefuroxime axetil is only available as a tablet (125, 250, and 500 mg), thereby limiting its usefulness in young children. Although the 125-mg tablets are small, they are very bitter tasting if crushed. Administration of cefuroxime axetil is associated with gastrointestinal toxicity similar in kind and frequency to that observed with amoxicillin/potassium clavulanate.

Cefixime is a third generation oral cephalosporin that is administered once daily. There has been no published study of the use of cefixime in patients with acute sinusitis. However, cefixime has been evaluated in the treatment of children with acute otitis media. Unfortunately, its activity against *S. pneumoniae* seems somewhat marginal although it is quite effective against β-lactamase producing *M. catarrhalis* and *H. influenzae* (13). Accordingly, it should be reserved for use in children in whom *S. pneumoniae* is no longer a suspected pathogen because of prior treatment with an agent such as amoxicillin, which is consistently active against *S. pneumoniae*.

One additional potential concern in selecting an antimicrobial regimen for patients with sinusitis is infection with anaerobes. However, these organisms are uncommon isolates in children with acute and subacute sinus infection (14). They should be considered in youngsters either with very protracted symptoms or those requiring surgical intervention. The gram-positive anaerobic streptococci and staphylococci are generally penicillin susceptible and therefore do not present a problem. Virtually all the therapeutic regimens discussed will be satisfactory. The gram-negative bacteroides species, which produce β-lactamase, should respond nicely to amoxicillin/potassium clavulanate.

DURATION OF THERAPY

Duration of antimicrobial therapy for patients with sinusitis has not been studied systematically. Empirically, a 10- to 14-day course of antimicrobials is recommended for patients with acute sinusitis. Most patients respond briskly to appropriate antimicrobials; cough and nasal discharge will improve in 48 to 72 h; if fever is present initially, it will diminish or resolve completely in the same time frame as will disturbances in appetite and sleep patterns. Accordingly, a 10-day regimen usually treats most patients for a week beyond the time at which they improve substantially or become symptom-free. If patients have not improved within 72 h of initiation of antimicrobials, an alternative agent should be selected.

If patients have improved slowly but are not yet asymptomatic by the tenth day of treatment, antimicrobial therapy should be extended for an additional 7 days. When patients present with very protracted symptoms, they often require longer courses of antimicrobial treatment. It may be a good rule of thumb to extend the course of antimicrobial therapy for 1 week beyond the time when symptoms have completely resolved in all patients with sinusitis. Hopefully, this will lead to complete eradication of bacterial colonization in a sinus mucosa that may not yet have been restored to normal.

RECURRENT SINUSITIS

Some children with acute sinusitis experience closely spaced recurrent infections. The most common risk factor for recurrent episodes of acute sinusitis is recurrent, closely spaced, viral upper respiratory infections. Contacts at day care centers or older siblings in the home may be the source of these recurrent viral infections.

Other risk factors or underlying problems to consider in patients with recurrent sinusitis are allergy, immunodeficiency of IgA with or without IgG-subclass deficiency, cystic fibrosis, immotile cilia syndrome, or anatomic abnormalities. One can readily screen for immunoglobulin deficiencies and cystic fibrosis. Except for allergy, often a difficult diagnosis to establish, the remaining problems are uncommon and, furthermore, not readily remediated.

Strategies for management of recurrent acute sinusitis have not been evaluated. Extrapolating from experience gained in the management of recurrent acute otitis media, it is tempting to consider antimicrobial prophylaxis for these patients. Criteria to be fulfilled prior to initiating antimicrobial prophylaxis might be similar to those frequently recommended for patients with recurrent otitis media; that is, three episodes of sinusitis in 6 months or four episodes in a year. This approach needs to be systematically evaluated in comparison to placebo. Selection of an antimicrobial agent for prophylaxis as well as duration of prophylactic treatment will likewise necessitate careful investigation.

ADJUNCTIVE THERAPY

Antihistamines, topical or oral decongestants, and anti-inflammatory agents have received little study in adults or children as adjunctive agents in the treatment of sinusitis. The role of antihistamines in the management of sinusitis in nonallergic children is controversial. In children with underlying allergy, antihistamines or topical therapy with steroids or cromolyn may be helpful. Phenylpropanolamine reduces symptoms of nasal congestion and objectively increases the diameter of the sinus ostia (15). However, oral decongestants can also cause thickening of secretions and thereby may have a potentially deleterious effect on their clearance from the sinus cavity. The use of topical decongestants may also cause relief of nasal symptoms but concern about rebound phenomena should limit their use. In addition, their net effect on the course of sinus infections is unknown.

Although the use of antibiotic therapy achieves a desirable therapeutic outcome in most patients, relapses and recurrences are common. Adjunctive therapies should be evaluated to determine if they can improve outcome in acute, subacute, or chronic disease.

REFERENCES

1. Wald ER, Reilly JS, Casselbrant M, et al. Treatment of acute maxillary sinusitis in childhood: a comparative study of amoxicillin and cefaclor. *J Pediatr* 1984;104:297–302.
2. Wald ER, Reilly JS, Casselbrant MC, Chiponis D. Treatment of acute sinusitis in children: Augmentin vs cefaclor. *Postgrad Med* 1984;Sept/Oct:133–136.
3. Wald ER, Chiponis D, Ledesma-Medina J. Comparative effectiveness of amoxicillin and amoxicillin–clavulanate potassium in acute paranasal sinus infections in children: a double-blind, placebo-controlled trial. *Pediatrics* 1986;77:795–800.
4. Rodriquez RS, De LaTorre C, Sanchez C, et al. Bacteriology and treatment of acute maxillary sinusitis in children: a comparative study of erythromycin–sulfisoxazole and amoxicillin. Abstracts of the Interscience Conference of Antimicrobial Agents and Chemotherapy (328) Los Angeles, CA, 1988.
5. Rachelefsky GS, Katz RM, Siegel SC. Chronic sinusitis in children with respiratory allergy: the role of antimicrobials. *J Allergy Clin Immunol* 1982;69:382–387.
6. Gwaltney JM, Sydnor A, Sande MA. Etiology and antimicrobial treatment of acute sinusitis. *Ann Otol Rhinol Laryngol* 1981;90(suppl 84):68–71.
7. Farr B, Scheld WM, Gwaltney JM, Sydnor A, Sande MA. Bacampicillin HCl in the treatment of acute maxillary sinusitis. *Bull NY Acad Med* 1983;59:477–481.
8. Scheld WM, Sydnor A, Farr B, Gratz JC, Gwaltney JM. Comparison of cyclacillin and amoxicillin for therapy of acute maxillary sinusitis. *Antimicrob Agents Chemother* 1986;30:350–353.

9. Sydnor AJ, Gwaltney JM Jr, Cochetto DM, Scheld, WM. Comparative evaluation of cefuroxime axetil and cefaclor for treatment of acute bacterial maxillary sinusitis. *Arch Otolaryngol Head Neck Surg* 1989;115:1430–1433.

10. Henderson FW, Gilligan PH. Wart K, Goff DA. Nasopharyngeal carriage of antibiotic-resistant pneumococci by children in group day care. *J Infect Dis* 1988;157:256–263.

11. Marchant CD, Shurin PA, Turczyk VA, et al. A randomized controlled trial of cefaclor compared with trimethoprim–sulfamethoxazole for treatment of acute otitis media. *J Pediatr* 1984;105:633–638.

12. Levine LR. Quantitative comparison of adverse reactions to cefaclor vs amoxicillin in a surveillance study. *Pediatr Infect Dis* 1985;4:358–360.

13. Howie VM, Owen MJ. Bacteriologic and clinical efficacy of cefixime compared with amoxicillin in acute otitis media. *Pediatr Infect Dis* 1987;6:989–991.

14. Wald ER, Byers C, Guerra N, Casselbrant M, Beste D. Subacute sinusitis in children. *J Pediatr* 1989;115:28–32.

15. Axelsson A, Jensen C, Melin O, et al. Treatment of acute maxillary sinusitis: amoxicillin, azidoillin, phenylpropanolamine and pivampicillin. *Acta Otolaryngol* 1981;91:313–318.

Pediatric Sinusitis,
edited by R. P. Lusk,
Raven Press, Ltd., New York © 1992.

CHAPTER 10

Surgical Management of Chronic Sinusitis

Rodney P. Lusk

The literature evaluating the surgical management of pediatric sinusitis is at best confusing. There is an increasing awareness that pediatric sinusitis is more common than once thought. Birrell (1) thought that sinusitis was underdiagnosed and reported that over a 5-year period only one case of acute maxillary sinusitis was diagnosed in over 10,000 examinations in the E.N.T. Department of the Royal Hospital for Sick Children in Edinburgh. There are few prospective studies evaluating any of the proposed methods of surgical management. This is due in part to the multifactorial nature of sinusitis and the difficulty in making the diagnosis. As we have seen in previous chapters, there are no signs or symptoms that are diagnostic of sinusitis. The severity of the disease cannot be predicted from the symptoms, and until recently we did not have a reliable method of staging the disease. Most of our assessments of severity of disease and symptoms are based on comparisons with plain sinus films, which we now know are inaccurate in assessing the extent and location of pediatric sinusitis (2).

Our current state of knowledge is lacking critical pieces of information that would allow us to ascertain the effect of our surgical modalities. We are unable to describe the prevalence or natural history of pediatric sinusitis. We do not have an accurate staging mechanism for pediatric sinusitis, and we have just started to understand how the disease vacillates.

The intent of this chapter is to discuss the existing methods of surgical management of pediatric chronic sinusitis and to indicate which of the methods remain viable options.

FOREIGN BODY

It is not rare in the pediatric population to have foreign bodies located within the nasal cavity. This will invariably present with purulent nasal discharge, nasal obstruction, and occasionally headache (Fig. 10.1). The foreign bodies are usually unilateral and therefore present with unilateral symptoms. Unilateral chronic sinusitis is very rare in this age group. These are particularly rewarding cases to treat as removal of the foreign body usually resolves the symptoms.

ADENOTONSILLECTOMY

Historical Perspective

Tonsil and adenoid hypertrophy may present with many of the same symptoms as chronic sinusitis. Previous investigations have shown an association be-

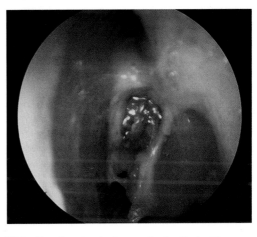

FIG. 10.1. Foreign body (a small plastic ball) presenting as chronic sinusitis.

R. P. Lusk: Department of Otolaryngology, St. Louis Children's Hospital, St. Louis, Missouri 63110.

tween children with "diseased" tonsils and adenoids and evidence of sinusitis. The incidence, however, varies widely with the methods of detection and the investigators. Almost all these studies are retrospective, and very few of them give any indication of duration of their follow-up.

Preston (3) found purulent rhinorrhea to be associated with tonsil and adenoid hypertrophy in 65% of children, and Wilson (4) found rhinorrhea in 27% of newborns. Indeed, it may be very difficult to differentiate between sinusitis and purulent rhinorrhea from other causes (5–7). There may also be a relationship between the size of the adenoids and the frequency of sinusitis (1,8,9). Merck (8) found that the size of the adenoid pad, as noted on lateral x-ray films, was related to a higher incidence of maxillary sinus abnormalities, noted on plain sinus films. Abnormal maxillary sinuses were noted in 13% of children with small adenoid pads, 24% with medium-sized adenoid pads, and 34% with large adenoid pads. Birrell (1) found that 27% of the 580 patients who underwent tonsillectomy and adenoidectomy had maxillary sinus infections as manifest by a positive antral puncture through the middle meatus. Similar results have been found by Mollison and Kendall (10) (22%), Crooks and Signy (11) (24%), and Gerrie (12) (9%). Carmack (13) attempted to rule out all patients with sinusitis or allergy and still found that 14.2% of the children undergoing "routine tonsillectomy and adenoidectomy" had positive findings on antral lavage. There appears to be an association between sinusitis and tonsil or adenoid disease, but the causal relationship remains unclear.

The role of tonsillectomy and adenoidectomy in treating sinusitis is also unclear. The early literature is supportive of tonsillectomy and adenoidectomy as a treatment modality, but the indications were not clearly defined in the articles (10,13–16). Stevenson (14) went so far as to say that he had never seen a case of maxillary sinusitis that did not have an adenoid pad present. Most of the papers seem to incriminate the adenoids as the source of the problem. Walker (17), however, found that the degree of infection of the tonsils was more of a factor than the size of the adenoid pad.

Griffiths (18), in 1937, states that "the indications are ill-founded for many tonsillectomies and adenoidectomies." The satisfactory results of tonsillectomy and adenoidectomy (T&A) have not been found to consistently correct chronic sinusitis (7,13,14,16,17,19). Paul (7) found that rhinorrhea, which was usually purulent and occurred in 84% of the patients, did not always clear after adenoidectomy and tonsillectomy. When the sinusitis was treated with antibiotics alone (for an unspecified time), he found that 11/50 cleared, 38/50 required antral lavage, and one required antrostomy. The success rate for T&A alone was only 18/

50, and 29/50 progressed to antral lavage. This study did not specify how long the patients remained asymptomatic, but it does reflect the inability of adenoidectomy alone to cure all sinusitis. Fujita et al. (20) evaluated the effect of adenoidectomy on sinusitis and eustachian tube function in 78 children 4 to 7 years old. He found that adenoidectomy "improved" nasal sinusitis in 56% of children, while 24% improved in the nonadenoidectomy group. He also found that in children with improved sinusitis, 73% had "active tubal function" while only 40% of the children with persistent sinusitis had "active tubal function." He concluded that patients who did not have sinusitis had better "tubal function."

The causal relationship between adenoid hypertrophy and sinusitis is not at all clear, but it would seem logical that if the adenoids were so large that there was stasis of secretions, then symptoms of sinusitis could be mimicked. The secretions could also cause inflammation of the sinus ostia to cause sinusitis. As Birrell (1) stated over 40 years ago, "no sinus can remain free from secretion when the nasal cavity, with which it communicates, contains a plentiful supply of secretion."

Recommendation

Our current state of knowledge does not allow us to predict whose sinusitis will resolve with adenoidectomy alone. It would seem prudent to examine the nasopharynx of the child to see if the adenoid pad or tonsils are so large that they cause stasis of secretions. If they are (Fig. 10.2), then performing an adenoidectomy, or tonsillectomy with adenoidectomy, may be a prudent first step. How large the adenoids must be before obstruction is present is a matter of judgment (Fig. 10.3). If they are not obstructive, our experience

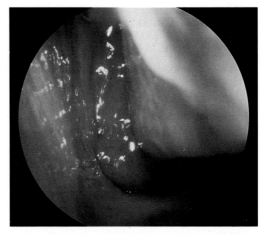

FIG. 10.2. Large obstructive adenoid pad causing symptoms compatible with sinusitis.

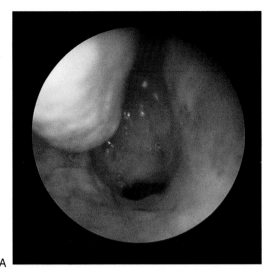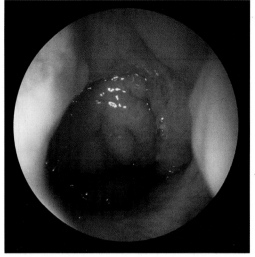

FIG. 10.3. A: Moderately large adenoid pad that could cause intermittent nasal obstruction and present with symptoms like sinusitis. **B:** Normal-sized adenoid pad.

indicates that the adenoidectomy does not effectively alter the course of the sinusitis.

One additional point must be made about the literature regarding adenoidectomy. Most of the studies relied on plain radiographs to diagnose maxillary sinus pathology. As indicated in the chapter on radiology by McAlister et al., we now know that the plain radiographs can be erroneous. Virtually all the authors who have addressed sinusitis equate sinus disease with maxillary sinus disease, and the ethmoid sinuses are not evaluated. We know that 23% of the patients who have clear maxillary sinuses will have ethmoid disease not detected on plain films (2). Until the advent of coronal CT scans, the status of ethmoid sinuses could not be accurately evaluated. It is likely that we shall find that maxillary sinus disease is more dependent on ethmoid disease than on adenoid hypertrophy.

ANTRAL LAVAGE

Historical Perspective

Infection of the maxillary sinus is difficult to detect by physical examination, signs, or symptoms (1,5,21). In the pediatric population the physical examination is accomplished with a head mirror, a microscope, an otoscope, or a telescope. Regardless of the method used, anterior rhinoscopy is all that can be accomplished in this age group.

The middle meatus is not well visualized. If there is no edema or secretions noted lateral to the middle turbinate, one can be encouraged but not assured that the osteomeatal complex is free of disease (Fig. 10.4). If purulence is seen in this region (Fig. 10.5), one cannot infer from the physical examination that the infection

FIG. 10.4. Normal entrance to the middle meatus without edema or purulence.

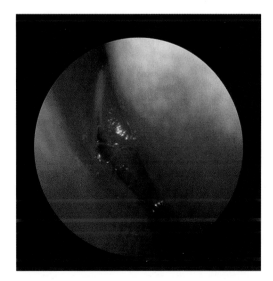

FIG. 10.5. Purulence in the superior middle meatus.

is isolated to the osteomeatal complex, or the anterior ethmoid, or the frontal or maxillary sinuses.

Infections of the sinuses are thought to originate in the nose (22–25). The epithelia of the nose and the sinuses are similar, and they are connected through the natural ostium of the sinus. A more detailed history of the pathophysiology of sinusitis is given in the chapter by Lusk and Wolf. During the acute infection, there may be stasis of secretions because of ciliary dyskinesia. Irrigation of the sinus is *not* thought to hasten recovery from acute maxillary sinusitis, and, in fact, the instrumentation may spread the infection into surrounding tissues (26). It is thought by some (27) that if the products of the infection are too thick to be transported through the natural ostium by the cilia, a persistent infection will occur and alter the mucosa of the sinus, in irreversible disease. The rationale for irrigation or lavage of the maxillary sinus is to suction or force debris out of the sinus through the natural ostium to promote reversal of the chronic sinusitis.

With the puncture, a hole can be placed in the sinus to examine it or to remove its contents by aspiration or irrigation. Both irrigation and sinusotomy are directed only to the maxillary sinus; it is not possible to irrigate the ethmoid or sphenoid sinuses. It is possible to perform trephination of the frontal sinus and irrigate it externally, but the frontal recess or duct is not easily cannulated, so only the external approach is practical. For these reasons the rather large body of literature involving lavage is directed only toward the maxillary sinus. This literature is therefore deficient in its assessment of chronic sinusitis because the therapy does not address other sinuses.

There are three methods of irrigating the maxillary sinus: through the natural ostium, through the inferior meatus, and through the canine fossa (anterior) puncture (Fig. 10.6).

1. Perhaps the oldest technique is through the natural ostium of the maxillary sinus. In the older patient, the procedure is usually performed under local anesthesia, unless it is combined with another procedure such as a tonsillectomy and/or adenoidectomy. The nose is anesthetized and vasoconstricted with 5% cocaine or a combination of lidocaine 4% and a topical vasoconstrictor such as 0.05% oxymetazoline or 0.025% phenylephrine. A curved cannula is then inserted into the middle meatus along the posterior half of the middle turbinate. The cannula is rotated laterally and pulled anteriorly to position it behind the uncinate process. With gentle lateral pressure, the cannula will engage the natural ostium, and, once in the ostium, the cannula is rotated laterally, inferiorly, and anteriorly. Then the maxillary sinus can be aspirated or lavaged with warm saline until clear.

The cannula cannot be introduced in all patients

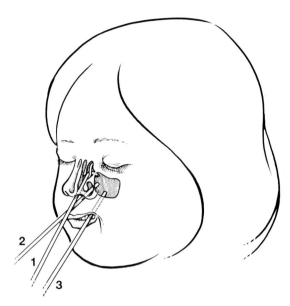

FIG. 10.6. Diagram depicting the three possible routes for maxillary sinus irrigation. (1) Through the natural ostium of the maxillary sinus. A curved suction-irrigator must be placed behind the uncinate process and engage the natural ostium. (2) Through the inferior meatus. This is limited by how well the floor of the maxillary sinus is developed. (3) Through the anterior wall of the maxillary sinus by going under the lip and through the gingival sulcus.

(28,29). Myerson (29) found that if the ostium was vertical, it could easily be entered, but if the ostium was horizontal it was more difficult to enter because of the deeper position in the lateral nose. The natural ostium is adjacent to the inferior and medial orbit, and the orbit can be entered accidentally if the surgeon is disoriented and forces the cannula through the lateral wall. It has been our experience that this is the region most likely to be penetrated during an ethmoidectomy. Once the irrigation is started, if the contents are clear, there is always a question about cannula placement and whether the irrigant is actually just going into the nose.

2. Lund (30) credits Gooch with the first description of an intranasal inferior meatal puncture in the 1770s. The procedure was not popularized until it was advocated by Lichtwitz (1886) (29), Krause (1887) (31), and Mikulicz (1887) (32). Mikulicz (32) preferred the inferior meatal puncture because (a) the middle meatal approach was not always anatomically possible, (b) there was a large blood vessel (spinopalatine) behind the middle turbinate that could result in troublesome bleeding, and (c) the natural ostium is in close proximity to the orbit, and penetration of the lamina papyracea could result in orbital complications. There was also concern about damage to the ostium of the maxillary sinus (33).

The inferior meatus is anesthetized with pledgets of topical anesthetic as previously described. If the procedure is performed under general anesthesia, vasoconstrictors are used to enhance visualization of the meatus. Inferior meatal puncture is accomplished through the inferior meatus with a straight sharp cannula (Lichtwitz). The cannula is positioned under the inferior meatus under direct visualization. This maneuver is greatly facilitated by using a Killian nasal speculum placed into the inferior meatus. Once contact is established with the meatal wall, the tip of the trocar is angled laterally as far as possible and rotated in a drilling manner to pierce the bone. Mollison and Kendall (10) suggest aiming for the lateral canthus of the eye, but we have found it useful to direct the trocar to the external canal of the ear. Once the trocar penetrates the bone, it slides in easily without resistance. The sinus should be first aspirated for air or fluid and then gently irrigated with warm saline. If blood is aspirated, it may mean that the trocar is located between the bone and the mucosal lining. If the sinus is not entered, the trocar should be repositioned and moved posteriorly (34). Air should not be injected back into the sinus for fear of causing an air embolism (35). With the inferior meatal approach, it is easier to assure oneself that the cannula is in the maxillary sinus; however, satisfactory anesthesia is more difficult to accomplish (26). This method has the additional disadvantage of not being useful in young children because the floor of the maxillary sinus has not developed below the insertion of the inferior turbinate.

Lavage has also been combined with the use of cannulas of different types for irrigating the maxillary sinus. Alden (36), Asherson (37), Carmack (13), and Stevenson (14) have recommended leaving in the antrum a cannula that comes out of the nose and can be used to irrigate the sinus several times a day. Huggill and Ballantyne (38) performed lavage in their evaluations and left a size 2 polyethene cannula in place and irrigated with a solution of 500 units/cc of penicillin. Over time these methods of treatment have proved unsuccessful and are now rarely used.

3. The canine fossa puncture is performed by going through the bone of the anterior antral wall. It is the most direct route to the sinus. It was originally introduced in 1743 and was repopularized in the early 1970s (39). Peterson thought this procedure easier and safer to perform under local anesthesia. Anesthesia is gained by infiltration into the gingival sulcus over the sinus with 1% lidocaine and 1:100,000 epinephrine. The infiltration is in a line under the pupil when the eye is in its neutral position inferior to the infraorbital foramen. The trocar is then inserted along the anesthetized path through the anterior wall of the maxillary sinus, taking care not to traumatize the infraorbital nerve. Once the trocar is in the sinus, the contents are aspirated and

irrigated as previously described. In the child this approach is likely the safest (26) but may be compromised by a high floor of the maxillary sinus, the potential of traumatizing the roots of the teeth, and a thick anterior wall. Ritter (26) feels the anterior approach is the safest, easiest, and the best endured by the patient. It is also easier to handle the endoscope, and the radius of action is the greatest (40). The examination of the ostium is significantly better through the canine approach, and bleeding is usually significantly less than with the inferior meatal approach.

In children the antrostomy for irrigation or sinoscopy can be difficult. A 3.0-mm trocar must be used with a 2.7-mm telescope. The anterior wall of the maxillary sinus is thicker and there is the real risk of traumatizing the roots of the permanent teeth. For this reason, Stammberger (41) does not recommend canine fossa puncture in children less than 9 years old. In children a canine fossa may be difficult to identify and the trocar will be guided by information gained on the coronal CT scan. A general anesthetic is required and a twisting motion is needed to push the trocar into the maxillary sinus. The maxillary sinus is smaller and more superior in children. The maxillary sinus is therefore harder to cannulate and increases the chance of creating false passages (Fig. 10.7). A false passage can be created into the nose by going through the middle meatus or the ostium. The trocar can be put into a tooth

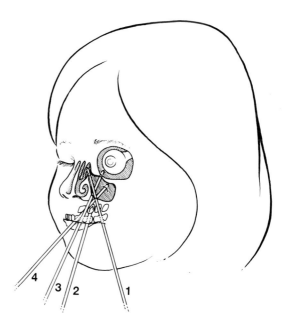

FIG. 10.7. Diagram of possible false passages created with the canine fossa approach: (1) through the medial wall of the sinus and into the middle meatus; (2) through the anterior wall and into a tooth bud; (3) through the roof of the maxillary sinus; and (4) through the posterior wall of the maxillary sinus and into the pterygopalatine fossa.

root with the sensation of falling into a cavity. The trocar can be passed through the roof of the maxillary sinus and into the orbit or through the posterior maxillary sinus wall. Finally, the trocar can be placed through the sinus and the posterior wall and into the pterygopalatine fossa. If these spaces are irrigated, significant complications can result.

Lavage has been combined with sinoscopy and has been used as a standard to measure the accuracy of plain radiographs. Kim et al. (40) report that the first effort to perform sinoscopy was in 1903 by Hirschmann through the canine fossa approach. Spielberg (42) adapted the inferior meatus approach to maxillary sinoscopy. Kim et al. (40) found that sinoscopy yielded the correct status of the maxillary sinusitis more frequently than did plain sinus films.

Objective Evidence

The effectiveness of the antral lavage has had mixed reviews in the literature. There have been many celebrated supporters of the intranasal lavage method of therapy. Carmack (13) recommended that lavage take place as early as possible and inferred that it should be used as a primary mode of therapy. Rarely, lavage will be successful with one intervention, and several authors (11,14,43,44) recommend multiple lavage before proceeding to a Caldwell–Luc procedure. Crooks and Signy (11) recommended weekly lavage until the patient was clear and reported as high as 10 lavage procedures before abandoning this mode of therapy. Alden (36) mentions that Dean administered general anesthesia (ethylene) to a child from six to twenty times in performing lavage for maxillary sinusitis. Stammberger (41) does not feel multiple lavages are necessary if adequate local decongestant is applied to the osteomeatal complex.

Recommendation

Antral lavage continues to be practiced today and in selected patients it has merit. There are no good prospective studies that allow us to make recommendations about which patients will respond to antral lavage. Inferior meatal lavage is traumatic, and it is not without potential complications. The canine fossa approach is perhaps easier, but adult patients frequently complain about the pain that sometimes persists. There is no reason to suspect that the pediatric patient is not equally predisposed to persistent pain. Most previous studies were performed before the use of prolonged antibiotic therapy, a mode of treatment that introduces additional variables, and lavage was required two to three times a week. In today's medical environment it is unlikely that parents, pediatricians, or otolaryngol-

ogists will tolerate local lavage at this frequency, and multiple general anesthetics will likely meet with equal resistance. Antral lavage, however, may be quite appropriate at the time of another procedure such as a tonsillectomy or adenoidectomy. Its overall efficacy requires further delineation.

INFERIOR MEATAL ANTROSTOMY

It is a natural progression of thought to treat failures of maxillary sinus lavage or irrigation by creating a larger hole in the sinus to allow better ventilation and drainage of the purulence.

Historical Perspective

The inferior meatal antrostomy has become the most popular surgical technique in the management of maxillary sinusitis (30) and therefore in the management of chronic sinusitis. In spite of its many advocates there has been little scientific investigation of its efficacy. As indicated with the lavage technique, the inferior meatal antrostomy was felt to be safer and technically easier than the middle meatal antrostomy (32). This procedure gained in popularity until introduction of the Caldwell–Luc procedure, which was preferred for several years and then became less popular. Lund (30) reports a steady decline in the incidence of inferior meatal antrostomy and Caldwell–Luc procedures at the Royal National, Throat, Nose and Ear Hospital from 1950 to 1985. There was a resurgence of the Caldwell–Luc procedure from 1979 to 1981 but a "marked" decrease since then.

Objective Evidence

A crucial factor in the success of the inferior meatal antrostomy is the patency of the "window" over time. Lund (30) did both a retrospective and prospective evaluation of inferior meatal antrostomy patency. In a retrospective evaluation of 216 patients, she found that 45% were closed, 50% were patent, and 5% could not be assessed. The age difference between the patent and the occluded groups was 35 years for the closed and 44 years for the patent antrostomies ($p = 0.05$). Of 15 patients younger than 16 years, 13 had closed antrostomies. The patent antrostomies were in patients 14 and 15 years old. A possible reason for the antrostomy closure is surgical technique, but the experience of the surgeon has not proved to be a significant factor (30). In a prospective study, Lund (30) created inferior meatal antrostomies from 2.5 to 5 cm in length and 1 to 5 cm in height. She found there was an initial loss of an average of 27% of the lumen over 5 weeks (which was the first time the lumen could accurately be measured). She concluded that the antrostomy had to be greater than 1 cm to remain patent. She also performed six antrostomies in four patients younger than 16, and all closed.

The inferior meatus is smaller in children than in adults, and it is therefore not possible to create an adequate-sized antrostomy. Patency in children appears to be difficult to achieve, and if patency is required for resolution of the sinusitis, one would expect a correspondingly low success rate in children. Muntz and Lusk (45) performed a retrospective evaluation of 39 children (mean age of 6.3 years) who had chronic sinusitis and had undergone bilateral inferior meatal antrostomies. They found a failure rate of 60% at 1 month and 73% at 6 months postoperatively. Seven of the patients had repeated inferior meatal antrostomies, with two improving and five failing.

The dependent position of the inferior meatal antrostomy was thought to improve drainage of the sinus and has been a cornerstone in the rationale for its use (46). It is now known that even though the sinus is ventilated, the mucociliary clearance patterns continue to transport the secretions to the natural ostium of the sinus (24,27,47). If there is obstruction at the ostium, secretions will accumulate and act as a source of infection. Indeed, the secretions can circulate from the nose through the inferior meatal antrostomy, into the maxillary sinus and up to the natural ostium (Fig. 10.8). The pooled secretions provide ample opportunity for bacterial replication.

Recommendation

As with antral lavage, there is little doubt that some patients and some children will benefit from inferior

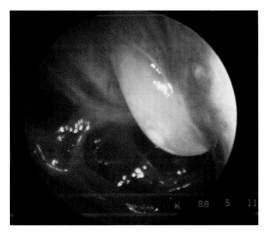

FIG. 10.8. Evidence of secretions being pulled from the nasal cavity into the maxillary sinus and transported to the maxillary ostium. (Photo provided by Dr. David Kennedy.)

meatal windows, but there are no prospective data available that would assist us in selecting the children who would benefit the most. The reasons for this include the inability to maintain patency, the high failure rate, and, in our estimation, other modalities, such as middle meatal antrostomy, that are less traumatic and more successful. We elected to abandon the procedure as a primary mode of therapy after reviewing our results (45). Currently, we have stopped using inferior meatal antrostomies to treat chronic sinusitis in children.

There is one exception, however. Children with ciliary dyskinesia do not have normal ciliary function, and in the subset of children with chronic sinusitis, inferior meatal antrostomies make sense, because gravity would be the primary means of evacuating secretions from the sinus. The problem of window patency, however, remains.

MIDDLE MEATAL ANTROSTOMY

Historical Perspective

Another mechanism for ventilating and draining the antrum is through the middle meatus and the natural ostium. Obstruction of the ostiomeatal complex has become a central theme in our current thinking about the cause of chronic sinusitis. As we have already noted, an early approach to irrigation of the sinus was through the natural ostium of the maxillary sinus. Around the turn of the century, Freer (48), Sluder (49), and Canfield (50) recommended removing most of the medial wall of the maxillary sinus through the middle and inferior meatus without removing the inferior turbinate. This aggressive management did not gain wide acceptance. Ostrum was cited by Wilkerson (51) as the first in the United States to forcefully make a case for limited middle meatal windows. This approach was thought to be technically more difficult and dangerous than the inferior meatus antrostomy (32). Proetz (33) felt that natural ostium should not be violated because the nerves and primary vascular supply came through the natural ostium (52). He felt the risk of protracted pain and paresthesia was high when the ostium was operated on. Hilding (53) performed a series of experiments creating maxillary antral windows at different sites in rabbits. Using three animals in each group, Hilding found that all three animals in which the natural ostium was widened became infected, whereas only two of three animals became infected when the opening was made in the inferior portion of the sinus. He also created an ostium as high on the medial wall as possible, as far from the natural ostium as possible, and none of the three animals became infected. Based on this work, Hilding recommended that an antrostomy should be as far from the natural ostium as possible. It was on the basis of this study that the concept of middle meatal antrostomy fell into disrepute (51). It should be noted in Hilding's defense, however, that he stated the following (53): "It cannot be concluded from these experiments that exactly the same results would occur in the sinuses of other species or in man." Wilkerson reports that the negative feelings against the middle meatal antrostomy were so strong that he stopped using it in spite of good results. He later returned to the approach and through his work (51) interest was rekindled in surgery in the middle meatus.

Objective Evidence

There has been little clinical research evaluating the effectiveness of middle meatal antrostomy. Kennedy et al. (27) retrospectively evaluated 117 antrostomies in 75 patients. In 20 procedures some surgical problems were encountered. In three the ostium could not be identified and in one, bleeding from the ethmoid cavity was a complicating factor. Of 95 procedures that had follow-up for greater than 4 months, 98% were patent. Two antrostomies were closed and four showed evidence of narrowing. Lavelle and Harrison (54) have reported a 94% patency rate in 150 patients undergoing intranasal middle meatal antrostomy over a 20-year period. Ninety-two percent of the patients in the series of Kennedy et al. (27) were asymptomatic or had significant improvement in their symptoms. The only complications reported were epiphora in two patients. Both occurred several months after surgery.

Recommendation

It appears that the middle meatal antrostomy carries a high patency rate. The approach allows removal of osteomeatal disease or anatomical abnormalities that may predispose the patient to have maxillary sinus disease. It retains the orientation of the mucociliary transport and physiologic drainage is reestablished. This approach has significant theoretical advantages and is a cornerstone in our current management of pediatric chronic sinusitis.

ENDOSCOPIC ETHMOIDECTOMY

External ethmoidectomy has been used to treat complicated sinus disease for a number of years. This approach gives maximum visualization and safety as the periosteum is retracted away from the ethmoid contents. Intranasal ethmoidectomy in the pediatric population has not been recommended by any authors because of the smaller size of the ethmoid cavity and the increased *potential* for complications. The transantral

approach to the ethmoid in children has not gained popularity because of fear of traumatizing the teeth. In addition, the anterior wall of the maxillary sinus is thick, and the sinus itself is small, which decreases the advantages of this approach. Because of these limitations, the endoscopic approach is particularly useful in children. It allows resection of disease in the ethmoid sinuses without scarring the face and has very little morbidity if the surgeon stays within the bounds of the ethmoid cavity.

Endoscopic ethmoidectomy in children is in its infancy, and the indications are just being defined. The failure of tonsillectomy, adenoidectomy, antral lavage, and inferior meatal windows to control symptoms of chronic sinusitis has lead to ethmoidectomy (partial or total) with maxillary antrostomy as a surgical treatment. This procedure appears to be safe in experienced hands but is not yet widely performed. Over the next several years, the technique will be modified and will evolve into a well-defined procedure.

The remainder of this chapter is directed toward the workup and surgical procedure for endoscopic ethmoidectomy.

Radiology

As indicated in the chapter by McAlister et al., the coronal CT scan has become a diagnostic cornerstone. We have found the axial scans to be of little use except in the sphenoid and possibly the frontal sinuses. The axial scan does not define the anatomy in a way that is useful to the surgeon. In the pediatric population, the sinuses are just developing and are difficult to accurately visualize. The plain films, unfortunately, both over- and under-read the amount of disease located in the ethmoid sinuses and cannot be used as a screening device to select children for a full CT scan. The reader is referred to the chapter by McAlister et al. for an indepth discussion of why we feel plain films are deficient. CT scans in the pediatric population are more difficult to perform because patients younger than 6 years usually require IV sedation. The CT scans are expensive and cannot be performed as frequently as the plain sinus films currently ordered by many pediatricians. As a matter of practicality, if the child's symptoms are severe enough and of sufficient duration that the surgeon and the parents would opt for surgical intervention, then it is reasonable to proceed with a CT scan. If the child is old enough to obtain a CT scan without sedation, then the indications may be more liberal.

It should be recalled that sinusitis is a disease that waxes and wanes and the CT scan cannot be used as the sole criterion for surgical intervention. Studies have not been performed correlating the CT scan results with the amount of disease seen at the time of surgical intervention. It is currently not possible to make any statements about the nature or the chronicity of the opacification seen in the sinuses on CT scans. In other words, opacification seen in the ethmoid cavities may be the result of an acute infection that will spontaneously resolve or chronic infection that is unlikely to clear without surgical intervention. Therefore a way to help differentiate the chronicity of the infection is to treat the patient with adequate medical therapy prior to performing the CT scan. We currently are using full-dose antibiotic therapy—amoxicillin/potassium clavulanate (Augmentin), erythromycin/sulfisoxazole (Pediazole), or cefuroxime-axetil (Ceftin)—and topical nasal steroid sprays for 4 weeks prior to obtaining the CT scan. There are no good prospective studies that define the efficacy of long-term antibiotic therapy or the use of topical nasal steroid sprays. It has been our experience that the use of topical beclomethasone has cleared the symptoms of a number of children. If disease is defined on the CT scan after appropriate therapy, *one cannot assume that the disease is irreversible and warrants surgical intervention.* The CT scans are one more factor to consider. If disease is present on CT scans but the patient is asymptomatic, then it is prudent to observe the patient without surgical intervention.

It is my belief that the CT scan accurately depicts the status of the sinuses on the day the study is obtained. I have had the experience of seeing disease limited to the anterior ethmoid complex on the CT scan and at the time of ethmoidectomy several weeks later, extensive disease was found in all the sinuses. The opposite has also occurred: the sinuses were completely opacified on CT scan but at the time of surgical intervention there was minimal disease. One has to look at the patient and the symptoms as a whole, and the CT scan is one additional piece of information to be considered.

Indications

Before the indications for the surgery are discussed, it is appropriate to discuss our current overall approach to the patient. Without doubt this approach will evolve and become refined as our knowledge of the disease process increases. It is our feeling that surgical intervention is undertaken after maximum medical management has failed. Maximum medical management has not been defined with prospective studies. If on initial evaluation there does not appear to be a good history or physical evidence of sinusitis, it is appropriate to reevaluate the child when he/she is ill to assess the signs and symptoms of disease. If the child has signs and symptoms compatible with sinusitis but has

not undergone an appropriate trial of medical management, it is appropriate to treat the patient with full-dose antibiotics and topical nasal steroid sprays for 4 weeks and then reassess. If the symptoms have been present for months or if there has not been resolution of symptoms with medical management, it is appropriate to proceed with a coronal CT scan. If the symptoms have been present for a few months and the response to medical management has been good, then a trial off antibiotics with maintenance topical nasal steroids is appropriate. The clinician uses his or her judgment to decide the best course of action. Although there are no studies evaluating the role of prophylactic antibiotics in sinusitis, I think this modality will be found to be important in the medical management of recurrent sinusitis.

If the CT scan shows no evidence of sinus disease, surgical intervention should not be undertaken; the patient should be managed with topical nasal steroid sprays and possibly antihistamines, although no prospective data are available on the effectiveness of either. It may be that prophylactic antibiotics are most efficacious in this setting. If the CT scan shows "pansinusitis," then surgical intervention will likely be warranted: however, it is not absolutely necessary because *we do not know the natural history of pediatric sinusitis* and therefore cannot predict with certainty the outcome of prolonged medical management. The hardest judgments to make are those regarding surgical intervention in children with minimal disease after prolonged medical management. As a general rule it is better to err on the conservative side: that is, when in doubt, it is best to continue medical management and follow the child's symptoms. With time, the best course will become clear. If the patient requires full-dose antibiotic therapy to remain free of disease, it is reasonable to consider surgery as an option.

Anesthesia

Surgical intervention in the pediatric population can be performed only under general anesthesia. As a general rule a thorough examination of the nose or ethmoid cavity is not possible in this age group because of poor compliance. In addition, cavity cleaning in the postoperative period is virtually impossible. For all practical purposes, any manipulation of the nasal cavity has to be under general anesthesia.

In our initial surgical procedures we used halothane and 4% cocaine but had some problems with arrhythmias and even some short runs of ventricular tachycardia. It was recognized that the halothane was probably sensitizing the myocardium to the cocaine, and once isoflurane was substituted the incidence of arrhythmias markedly decreased. A more extensive dis-

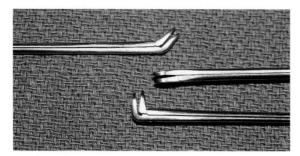

FIG. 10.9. Pediatric cup forceps.

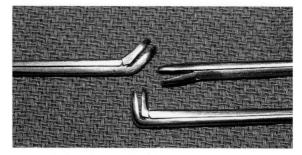

FIG. 10.10. Adolescent cup forceps.

cussion of the anesthesia is presented in this chapter under the section on vasoconstriction.

Instrumentation

It is imperative to use the right instrumentation in children if the risks of complications are to be minimized. When I first performed pediatric ethmoidectomies, appropriate instrumentation was not available. The adult instruments were much too large to be safely used in children, so middle ear instruments were used. These were not designed for the task and were generally too short to work effectively in the posterior ethmoid sinus. Later, with Karl Storz, we designed a set of instruments for pediatrics. The cups are based on the same design as the adult Blakesly forceps and come in two sizes, pediatric (Fig. 10.9) and adolescent (Fig. 10.10). The adolescent forceps is best used in children older than 8 years and is becoming the preferred instrument by some surgeons for adult ethmoidectomies. Pediatric suction forceps have also been designed (Fig. 10.11) and are advantageous if there is any significant bleeding. Because of the narrowness of the small child's nose, the suction forceps may be difficult to use with a 4-mm or even a 2.7-mm telescope.

An instrument that is unique to the pediatric set is the seeker (Fig. 10.12). This instrument is used to identify the natural ostium of the maxillary sinus and to infracture the medial wall of the maxillary sinus. It has a narrow ball on one tip and a wider one on the other. In smaller children the narrow end is easiest to use, but it must never be forced into the ostium. The narrow end can also be used to gently probe the hiatus semilunaris, the frontal recess, or the sinus lateralis. It is also an excellent instrument for manipulating small fragments of bone from the ethmoid roof and frontal recess.

The pediatric set also contains a curette fashioned after the J curette used in ears. The curette is longer than the ear instrument, and the other end has a 90-degree bend (Fig. 10.13) that is used in the agger nasi cells and in the anterior portion of the natural ostium of the maxillary sinus. The J curette is used to enter anterior and posterior ethmoid cells in a controlled manner.

The telescopes used are the 2.7- and 4.0-mm Hopkins rod-lens telescopes. In general, one should use the larger scope to permit better lighting and visualization (Fig. 10.14A). The smaller scopes provide a considerably smaller image, and there is less light (Fig. 10.14B). The beginning pediatric endoscopist should make every effort to use the larger telescope to increase the field of view and provide as much illumination as possible. With experience the 2.7-mm telescope will become more comfortable and can be used safely. Not infrequently, the 2.7-mm telescope will have to be used to perform the uncinectomy, and the

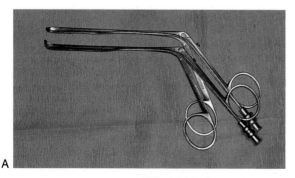

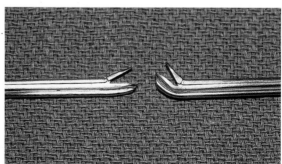

FIG. 10.11. Pediatric cup forceps with suction attached.

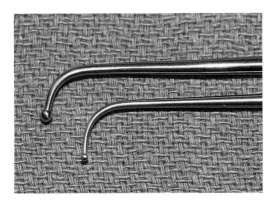

FIG. 10.12. Curved instrument used as a seeker to palpate the maxillary sinus ostium, frontal recess, and sinus lateralis.

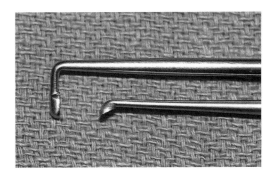

FIG. 10.13. J curette with straight and 90-degree ends.

larger scope can be used in the ethmoid cavity. Varying angles of telescopes are available, but most surgery is performed with the 0-degree telescope. The 30-degree telescope is useful in enlarging the maxillary ostium, examining the maxillary sinus through the ostium, identifying the lamina papyracea, and working in the frontal recess. The 70-degree telescope is difficult to use in children and should not be used with forceps unless the surgeon is very experienced. This scope is best positioned through a trocar, which has been previously placed with a 0- or 30-degree telescope.

Surgical Technique

Surgery of the pediatric sinuses cannot be performed safely without a thorough knowledge of the anatomy of the nose. An extensive discussion of the lateral nasal anatomy is not presented here because there are ex-

cellent articles and books on this subject (41,55–57). Anatomical landmarks of special importance in the pediatric population are discussed in the chapter by Muntz and Lusk. Figure 10.15 is an axial diagram of the middle turbinate and the mid-anterior ethmoids. This diagram is used to help explain the surgical procedure. It is important to note that all the anatomical structures are present in the pediatric population, but the ethmoid labyrinth is smaller than in the adult, and the surgery therefore must be precise, with careful identification of all landmarks.

As a basic principle I think surgery in children should be as conservative as possible while correcting the underlying problem. In some children this may require only opening the infundibulum (although in our experience this is rare), while others will require anterior and posterior ethmoidectomy and maxillary antrostomy. Disease in the pediatric age group is located primarily in the anterior ethmoid and maxillary sinuses (2). Stammberger (22,24,58) notes that the anterior ethmoid, especially the infundibulum, holds the key to recurrent sinusitis.

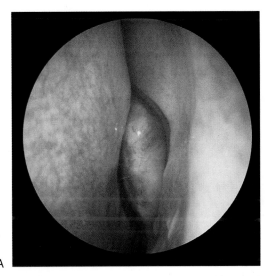
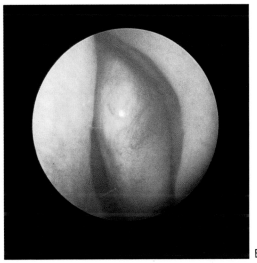

FIG. 10.14. A: View with a 4-mm Hopkins rod telescope. **B:** View with a 2.7-mm Hopkins rod telescope.

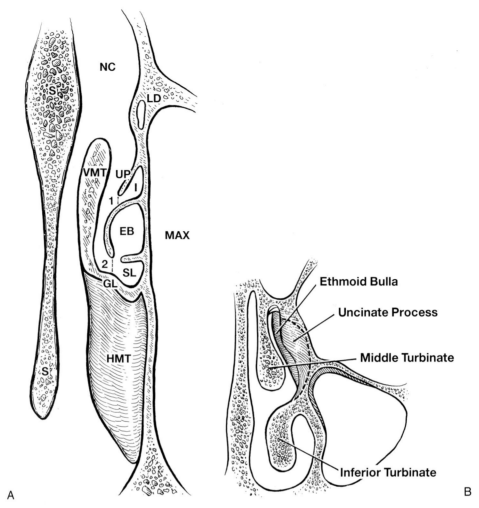

FIG. 10.15. A: Schematic drawing of the middle turbinate and the anterior ethmoid cells. NC, nasal cavity; LD, lacrimal duct; VMT, vertical middle turbinate; UP, uncinate process; I, infundibulum; EB, ethmoid bulla; SL, sinus lateralis; GL, ground (basal or grand) lamella; HMT, horizontal lamella; S, septum; MAX, maxillary sinus; 1, inferior hiatus semilunaris; 2, superior hiatus semilunaris. **B:** Coronal drawing of the anatomy at the uncinate process.

As Rice and Schaefer have noted, the endoscopic techniques developed in Europe by Messerklinger and Wigand were for disease at two ends of the spectrum: the Messerklinger technique (57,59) for early anterior ethmoid disease and the Wigand technique (56,60–62) for pansinusitis or in patients in whom the more conservative procedure is apt to fail. Since we know that in the majority of children the disease is located in the anterior ethmoid and maxillary sinuses, I have adopted the Messerklinger technique, which has been so carefully clarified by Stammberger (22–24,63) and Kennedy (25,27,64,65). This approach addresses the disease at its early stages and removes only the diseased tissue and leaves as much normal anatomy as possible. Radical sphenoidectomies can be performed using these principles; however, it is not frequently necessary in children.

Regardless of the technique, intranasal endoscopic surgery has two goals: (a) maximal preservation of all normal mucosa and (b) to secure communication between the nasal cavity and the paranasal sinuses via the natural channels to promote free drainage and aeration of the cavity (56). This does not require removal of all the cells or mucosa but does require opening the areas of obstruction. As Wigand states (56), intranasal endoscopic operations on the paranasal sinuses for chronic sinusitis are mainly limited to opening the narrow bony points to restore ventilation and internal drainage. The operation therefore should be tailored to the individual patient and the extent of the chronic sinusitis.

I have tried to standardize the approach as much as possible in an effort to minimize the risk of complications and yet perform an adequate operation. The following description is the method I currently am using. It has proved to be safe and is proving efficacious in the training of pediatric otolaryngology fellows performing ethmoid surgery.

Preparation of Patient and General Comments

A general anesthetic is always used in children. The child may initially be induced with halothane, but it is our recommendation that halothane be stopped before vasoconstriction is started.

The patient should be intubated with an endotracheal tube large enough to have leak greater than 15 cm H_2O. If not, the leak increases during the case, exposing the surgeon to anesthetic gases and increasing the difficulty of the surgery because blood coats the end of the telescope on each expiration. A snug fit with the endotracheal tube is not a problem. Once the patient is intubated, the nose is vasoconstricted as noted below.

The patient's head is rotated toward the surgeon, the head end of the bed is elevated approximately 30 degrees above the thorax, and the neck is extended approximately 15 degrees (Fig. 10.16).

The head is wrapped with a towel, but the eyes are not covered. Lacrilube or some similar agent is placed on the cornea to prevent it from drying. Particular care must be used when passing instruments across the head to prevent dropping objects on the face or in the eyes.

The position of the operating room personnel and equipment is variable and the setup that I use is diagramed in Fig. 10.17. The surgeon is seated at the right side of the patient with the legs comfortably positioned under the shoulders. The left arm is best rested on a Mayo stand or table. The left hand is used to hold the telescope and it is best to look through the scope with the left eye and close the right eye. With practice, the image in the right eye can be suppressed so the eye

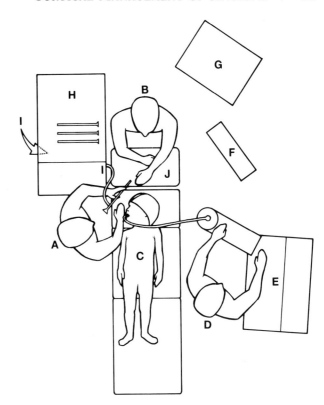

FIG. 10.17. Positions of personnel and equipment in the operating room. A, Surgeon; B, nurse; C, patient; D, anesthetist; E, anesthesia machine; F, x-ray view box; G, monitor and VHS recorder; H, back table for infrequently used instruments; I, light sources under table; J, Mayo stand for frequently used instruments.

doesn't have to be closed. The right eye is opened and used to pass instruments into the nose. This minimizes the chance of traumatizing the nasal mucosa.

The CT scan should be positioned directly across from the surgeon to allow frequent reference (Fig. 10.11). The surgeon and nurse should gown, glove, and mask for their protection. The position of the nurse is a matter of personal preference; however, we have found it most convenient for the nurse to be located at the head of the patient. On the nurse's table is a pan with normal saline in which all the specimens are placed. The nurse should immediately inform the surgeon if tissue floats. There are three types of tissue that float: (a) mucosa, which is the most common and has air trapped within, (b) orbital fat, and (c) brain. We place the light sources on the bottom shelf of the table under the left elbow. This allows the light source to be close to the patient and provides maximum flexibility and length of the light cords.

If a video monitor is used, we find it best positioned to the nurse's left and in front of the surgeon. My instructing experience at courses has taught me the importance of spatial orientation. Students invariably

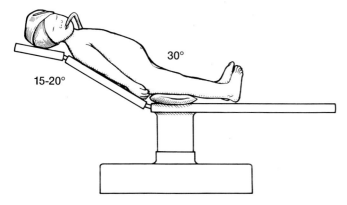

FIG. 10.16. Position of the patient on the operating table.

have more difficulty with coordination and orientation when trying to operate off the monitor. We therefore recommend using a beam splitter and looking through the scope rather than looking at a monitor. This is especially true for the tight spaces encountered in the pediatric nose.

Application of Vasoconstriction

We evaluated three different vasoconstricting agents during functional endoscopic sinus surgery (FESS) in 57 children. Oxymetazoline 0.05%, phenylephrine 0.25%, or cocaine 4% was applied to the nasal mucosa in a prospective, randomized, double-blind fashion. The surgeon's subjective impressions of bleeding and visualization were recorded for each side of the nose, as were total blood loss and anesthesia time. While all three vasoconstrictors were tolerated well by the children, subjective scoring for bleeding showed that children receiving oxymetazoline 0.05% were less likely to receive scores of "more" bleeding than usual (3/38 versus 10/34 for phenylephrine 0.25% and 10/35 for cocaine 4%, $p < 0.02$). Subjective scoring for visualization showed that children receiving oxymetazoline 0.05% were also *less* likely to receive scores of "worse" visualization than usual (3/38 versus 12/38 for phenylephrine 0.25% and 9/35 for cocaine 4%, $p < 0.01$). There was no difference in surgical bleeding or visualization between children receiving phenylephrine and children receiving cocaine. In our institution, 0.05% oxymetazoline (A) is the preferred vasoconstrictor for FESS in children. Two patients in the 0.25% phenylephrine group had the surgical procedure aborted because of bleeding severe enough to compromise visualization.

We prefer to apply vasoconstrictors on ½-in. neuropledgets (Fig. 10.18). The pledgets are initially applied to the anterior nose for 5 min and then removed. This has to be performed with great care as traumatized septal mucosa will cover the lens of the scope from that point on. This error converts any procedure into a difficult one. I have found it best to first vasoconstrict one side and then, as this side is finished, the opposite side is vasoconstricted. It is my impression

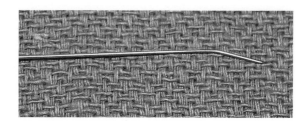

FIG. 10.19. A number 25-gauge spinal needle bent toward the bevel and used for injection.

that if both sides are vasoconstricted at the beginning there is a rebound vasodilation on the second side resulting in decreased visualization and increased intraoperative bleeding. This has not, however, been examined in a prospective manner.

Injection of Local Anesthetic

A number 25-gauge spinal needle is bent at the tip approximately 5 to 10 degrees toward the bevel and attached to a 3-cc syringe (Fig. 10.19). An injection of 1% lidocaine with 1/100,000 epinephrine is placed first, under direct visualization, posterior to the ethmoid bulla along the basal lamella (Fig. 10.20). This injection is intended to block the peripheral branches of the sphenopalatine artery. Two additional injections are placed along the uncinate process (Fig. 10.21). The top injection is placed just below the juncture of the middle turbinate. The injection is started with gentle pressure just under the mucosal surface. Pressure equivalent to that used in the posterior superior quadrant of the middle ear will be necessary. Frequently, the needle is pushed too hard and it will go into the infundibulum

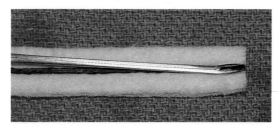

FIG. 10.18. Position of alligator grasping a ½-in. neuropledget.

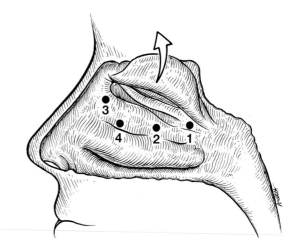

FIG. 10.20. Injection sites for ethmoidectomy: 1, inferior basal lamina; 2, inferior uncinate process; 3, superior uncinate process; 4, occasionally anterior to the uncinate process.

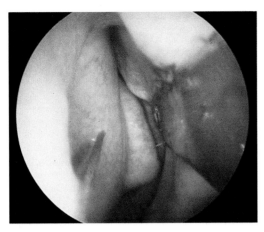

FIG. 10.21. A number 25-gauge spinal needle injecting the uncinate process.

(Fig. 10.22). When this happens, the local will infiltrate into the infundibulum and not under the mucosa and subsequent injections are difficult. Occasionally, additional injections anterior to the uncinate process are used if significant blanching has not been noted (Fig. 10.20). Two pledgets of 0.05% oxymetazoline are placed into the nose, taking care to place the first into the middle meatus along the uncinate process. If the pledgets are forced into the middle meatus, the lateral surface of the middle turbinate will be traumatized with resultant increased bleeding and risk of scarring. These pledgets are left in place for another 5 to 7 min.

Inspection of Nasal Cavity

After the nose has been adequately vasoconstricted, it is examined with a 0-degree 2.7-mm telescope. The first pass is along the floor of the nose, and the size of the adenoid pad is examined. Any purulence in the

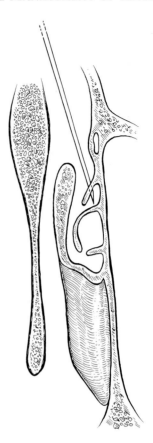

FIG. 10.22. Diagram of the needle being thrust too deep into the infundibulum (anatomy based on Fig. 10.15A).

nose is carefully suctioned, and its apparent source is a valuable indicator of the sinus involved. If the purulence is present only in the nose, it will be rapidly and easily suctioned from the nasal cavity. If the secretions are thick, tenacious, and from the middle meatus, they are likely to be coming from the maxillary sinus (Fig. 10.23). If it is coming from the medial side

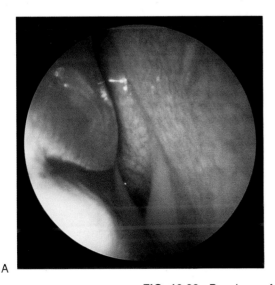

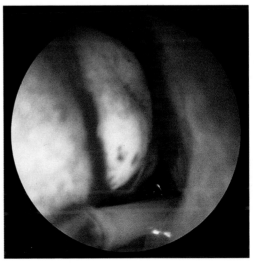

A

B

FIG. 10.23. Purulence from the maxillary sinus.

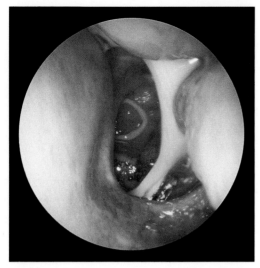

FIG. 10.24. Purulence from the superior meatus and sphenoid recess.

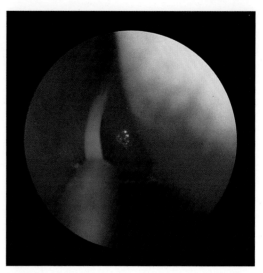

FIG. 10.25. Purulence from the superior middle meatus and the frontal recess.

of the middle turbinate, its source is the superior meatus (posterior ethmoid cells) or the sphenoid sinus (Fig. 10.24). Purulence from the root of the middle meatus is likely originating from the frontal sinus or agger nasi cells (Fig. 10.25).

Usually an obstructive adenoid pad would have already been noted and the decision about adenoidectomy would have been made preoperatively. Examination of the sphenoid recess in children is difficult even for the 2.7-mm telescope because of the very narrow channel and inadequate vasoconstriction. If there is reason to examine this area, it is best accomplished after the anterior ethmoidectomy because the middle turbinate is easier to displace laterally, which gives better exposure to the recess.

It is difficult to roll the scope under the middle turbinate and into the middle meatus as is done in adults (Fig. 10.26). I have found medial retraction of the mid-

dle turbinate with a Freer elevator to be an effective way of examining the anterior middle meatus. In this way the uncinate is examined and the medial edge of the ethmoid bulla is frequently noted (Fig. 10.27).

The following is a description of the endoscopic ethmoidectomy as I currently practice it.

Incision into the Uncinate Process (Basal Lamella 1)

Clear identification of the uncinate process is essential to appropriately place the incision and to reduce the risk of entering the orbit. Identification of the uncinate process is perhaps the most crucial step in the operation. The uncinate process can be identified in all cases except those of the hypoplastic maxillary sinus (Fig. 10.28). The hypoplastic sinus can clearly

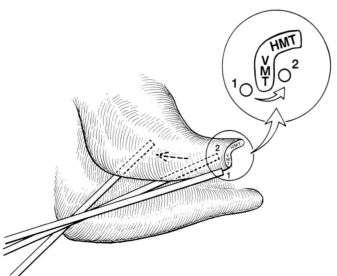

FIG. 10.26. Diagram of the scope rolled into the middle meatus. (HMT, horizontal middle turbinate; VMT, vertical middle turbinate.)

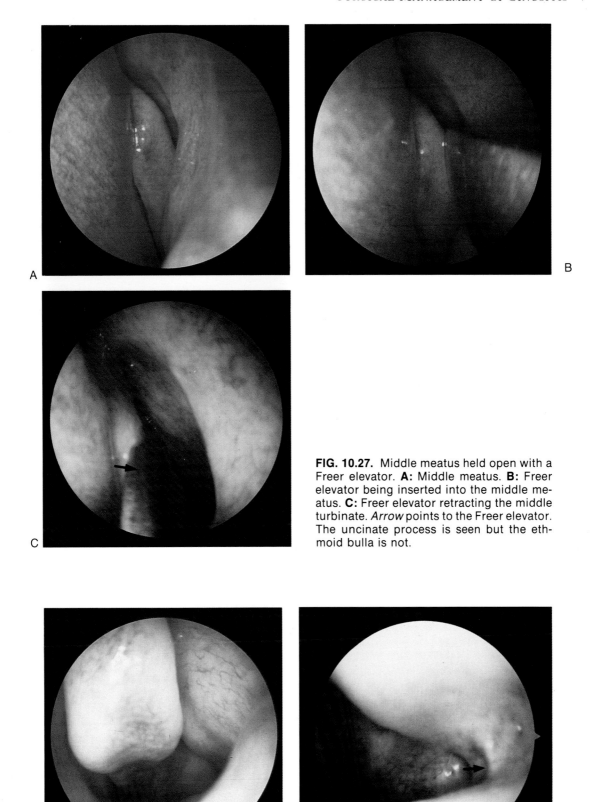

FIG. 10.27. Middle meatus held open with a Freer elevator. **A:** Middle meatus. **B:** Freer elevator being inserted into the middle meatus. **C:** Freer elevator retracting the middle turbinate. *Arrow* points to the Freer elevator. The uncinate process is seen but the ethmoid bulla is not.

FIG. 10.28. Endoscopic view of hypoplastic maxillary sinus. **A:** Examination of the middle meatus with a 0-degree telescope. **B:** Examination of the obstructed ostium with a 30-degree telescope. *Arrow* points to the obstructed ostium.

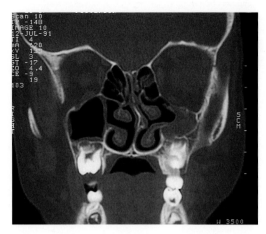

FIG. 10.29. Coronal CT scan of hypoplastic maxillary sinus.

be identified on coronal CT scans (Fig. 10.29). The position of the uncinate is relatively constant in children, but significant variation can occur (see chapter by Muntz and Lusk). It is a good idea to palpate the structure that is thought to be the uncinate process. If the uncinate is correctly identified, it will move slightly laterally when palpated with a Freer elevator or a similar instrument (Fig. 10.30). Careful visualization of the lateral border will show a "break point" where the uncinate process hinges with the lateral wall of the nose.

The seeker can be used to palpate the hiatus semilunaris and the tip can "pull" the uncinate medially to even further identify the uncinate process (Fig. 10.31). The incision is performed just medial to this break point (Figs. 10.32 and 10.15B). If the break point is not

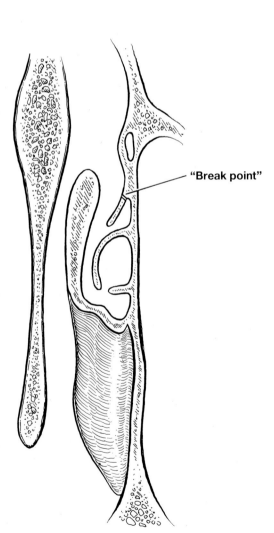

FIG. 10.30. Diagram of the "break point" of the uncinate process.

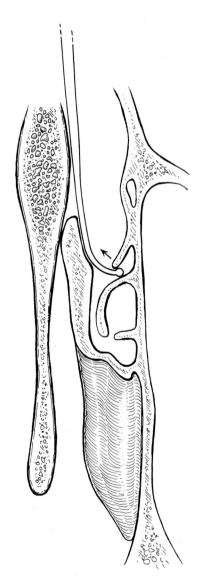

FIG. 10.31. Diagram of the small end of the seeker being inserted into the hiatus semilunaris and "pulling" the uncinate anteriorly.

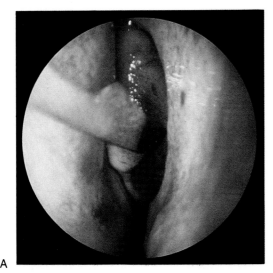

A

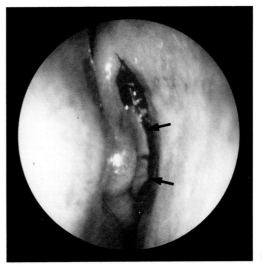

B

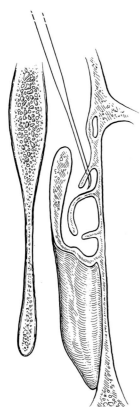

C

FIG. 10.32. Incision into the uncinate process with a sickle knife. **A:** Incision frequently has to be made without direct visualization. **B:** Incision of the uncinate process completed (*arrows*) but the uncinate process has not been removed. **C:** Diagram of the ideal incision site. Also refer to Fig. 10.15B.

clearly identified, it is best to remove the uncinate process in strips starting medially along the posterior border or with a back-biting forceps.

On occasion an accessory ostium can be noted in the uncinate process (Fig. 10.33A–D). This provides a view into the undisturbed infundibulum. On occasion the natural ostium to the maxillary sinus can be seen through the accessory ostium (Fig. 10.33C,D). Kennedy and Stammberger have recommended performing the incision from superior to inferior, but I have

found it easier to proceed from inferior to superior in children. The uncinate process is smaller and thinner than in the adult; therefore the incision should be made carefully to prevent incising the ethmoid bulla or lamina papyracea. Curved sickle knives should be used with great care because they increase the chance of incising the lamina papyracea. The incision is started along the posterior margin and is carried superiorly to the thicker bone adjacent to the root of the middle turbinate. The incision is terminated below the root of

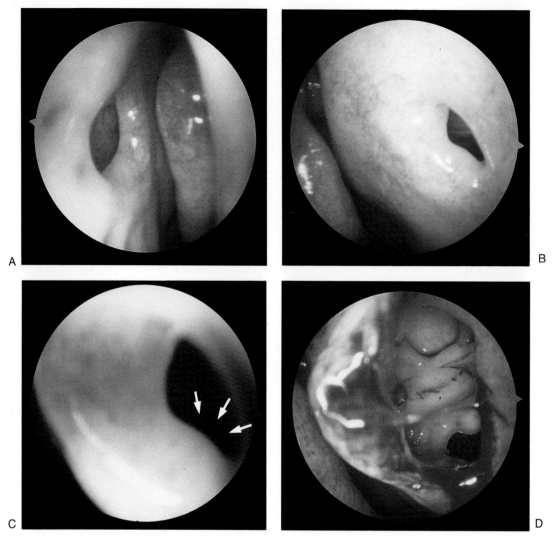

FIG. 10.33. View of bilateral accessory ostia of the uncinate process. **A:** Right uncinate accessory ostium and infundibulum. **B:** Left uncinate accessory ostium and infundibulum. **C:** Close-up view through the accessory ostium into the infundibulum; the ostium to the maxillary sinus can be seen as a dark hole. **D:** After the incision into the uncinate process has been performed the ostium to the maxillary sinus is clearly identified.

the middle turbinate (Fig. 10.34). This will prevent the mucosa from tearing onto the middle turbinate and decrease the chance of scarring. If the incision into the middle meatus is not clean, a pair of scissors can be used to transect the mucosa.

A pediatric straight-biting forceps is rotated to allow the nonmobile jaw to retract the middle turbinate medially and to grasp the incised uncinate process (Fig. 10.35).

Once the uncinate process is engaged, the forceps is closed and rotated. It is best to grasp the uncinate process first inferiorly and then superiorly. If the mucosa is stripping onto the middle turbinate superiorly, the maneuver is stopped and the scissors are used to incise the mucosa before the uncinate process is removed. Once the uncinate process is removed, a J curette is used to remove any residual uncinate bone at

its lateral attachment. It is crucial to make sure that all the uncinate is removed to improve access to the middle meatus, prevent scarring, and prevent a narrowed middle meatus postoperatively (see Fig. 10.76C). Wigand (56) has stated that simple enlargement of the semilunar hiatus by resection of the upper edge of the uncinate process should be termed a *hiatotomy* while an *infundibulotomy* indicates a wide opening of the ethmoid infundibulum with removal of the ethmoid bulla.

On occasion, even in the pediatric age group, a concha bullosa will be present and cause enough obstruction that the procedure cannot be performed (Fig. 10.36A). In this case the lateral half of the middle turbinate can be incised (Fig. 10.36B) and removed (Fig. 10.36C). Exposure to the uncinate process and the middle meatus is then easily accomplished.

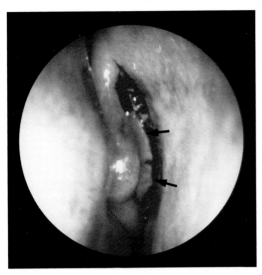

FIG. 10.34. Incision terminated below the root of the attachment of the middle turbinate. Mucosa is left intact along the line noted by the *arrows*.

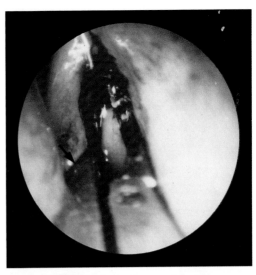

FIG. 10.35. Straight pediatric cup forceps are used to remove the uncinate process. The fixed (nonmobile) portion of the cup (*arrow*) is used to gently retract the middle turbinate medially.

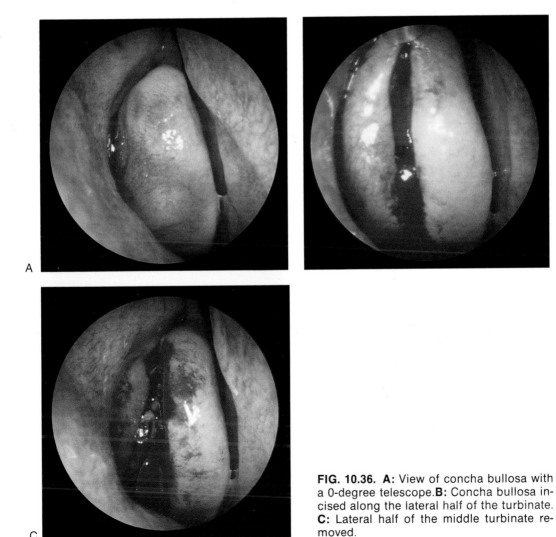

FIG. 10.36. **A:** View of concha bullosa with a 0-degree telescope. **B:** Concha bullosa incised along the lateral half of the turbinate. **C:** Lateral half of the middle turbinate removed.

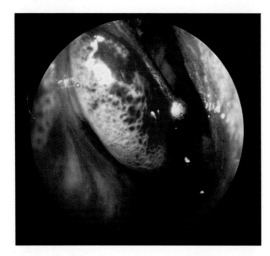

FIG. 10.37. Seeker retracting the middle turbinate to allow insertion of the 30-degree telescope.

Maxillary Ostium

Most adult surgeons recommend waiting until the ethmoidectomy has been performed before addressing the natural ostium of the maxillary sinus. At the urging of Dr. Parsons from San Antonio, I have started identifying and examining the ostium immediately after performing the uncinectomy. It is now my impression that the ostium is easiest to identify and enlarge at the beginning of the procedure because the bleeding is less, and with a 30-degree telescope the size of the ostium and the degree of obstruction can most accurately be assessed. If the ostium is obvious and not obstructed, it should not be enlarged. If it is not clearly seen, a seeker is used to identify it. The curved neck of the seeker retracts the turbinate (Fig. 10.37), the 30-degree scope is advanced into the middle meatus, and the small end of the seeker is inserted into the space behind the posterior mucosal surface of the uncinate process (Fig. 10.38). A frequent error is to place the seeker into the area where the uncinate bone has been removed. The seeker should be forced into the maxillary sinus only as a last resort because forcing it frequently will strip the maxillary mucosa from the roof of the sinus and create a false passage (Fig. 10.39).

Once in the ostium, the tip of the seeker is rotated inferiorly and the neck is forced medially and inferiorly (without rotation of the tip) to medially displace the inferior margin of the ostium (Fig. 10.40). Usually several bubbles will be seen coming through the ostium of the maxillary sinus if the fontanelle is pressed laterally. If the fontanelle is opened instead of the natural ostium, not infrequently the mucosa will be stripped from the posterior wall of the maxillary sinus (Fig. 10.41). If the mucosa has stripped off the roof of the sinus, it is very difficult to find the natural ostium and further attempts to penetrate the mucosa with the seeker will only increase the size of the false passage. I have found it easiest to incise the mucosa with a sickle knife and carry the incision into the posterior fontanelle with the scissors. Stammberger (41) has noted that a sucker can be used to pull the mucosa back into its normal position. I have found this to be a very helpful maneuver in children. If the ostium is

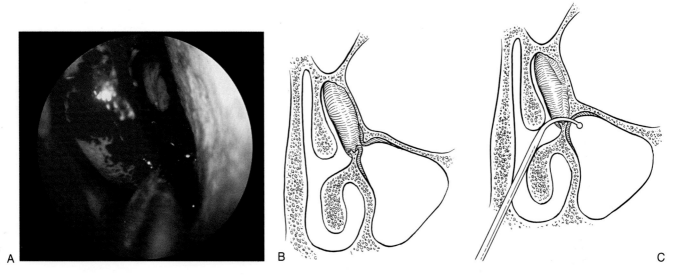

FIG. 10.38. A: The seeker is used to palpate and cannulate the natural ostium of the maxillary sinus. Here the seeker is inserted into the ostium of the maxillary sinus. **B:** Diagram of natural ostium after the uncinate process has been removed. **C:** Diagram of seeker entering the maxillary sinus through the natural ostium.

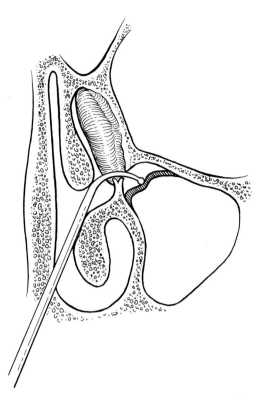

FIG. 10.39. Diagram of the seeker stripping the mucosa from the roof of the maxillary sinus.

to be enlarged, the posterior fontanelle is best opened through the natural ostium with a pair of scissors (Fig. 10.42). The scissors are rotated to allow the upper moving blade to be inserted through the ostium into the maxillary sinus. An attempt is made to curve the posterior surface of the incision inferiorly. Next, the back-biting forceps is placed into the middle meatus

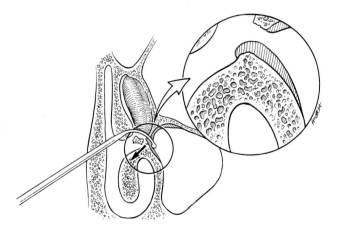

FIG. 10.40. Diagram depicting the movement of the seeker to open the ostium of the maxillary sinus: (1) the seeker is inserted into the ostium; (2) the seeker is rotated inferiorly then (3) pushed medially to infracture the remaining uncinate process.

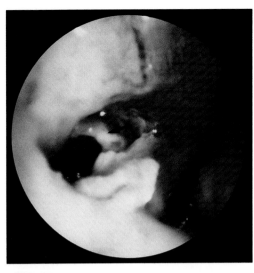

FIG. 10.41. The *arrow* shows the mucosa that can be stripped from the roof and the posterior maxillary wall if the maxillary ostium is not entered.

by running it along the floor of the nose and then rotating it up and into the middle meatus (Fig. 10.43A). This maneuver retracts the middle turbinate and allows good visualization of the ostium. A portion of the anterior fontanelle is removed, taking care not to extend the incision into the lacrimal duct (Fig. 10.43B).

Karl Storz makes three "back-biters." The thinnest with the short jaw is the only one satisfactory for pediatric work (Fig. 10.43A). The back-biter is advanced posteriorly until the jaw can be opened and the instrument placed atraumatically into the ostium. The longer jaws are not satisfactory in children because the end of the instrument hits the basal lamella before the jaw can be opened into the ostium. Then the back-biter is pulled forward to just engage the anterior portion of the ostium. Care must be taken in children not to take

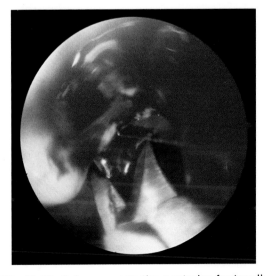

FIG. 10.42. Scissors open the posterior fontanelle.

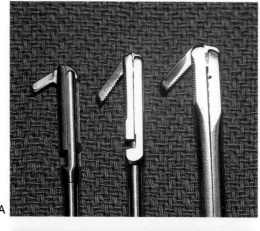

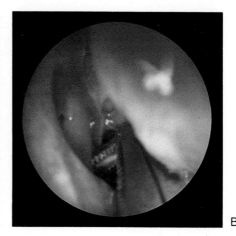

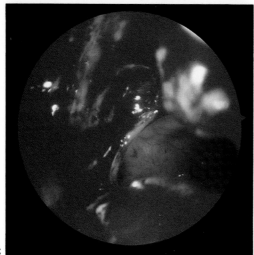

FIG. 10.43. A: Three sizes of back-biting forceps available from Karl Storz. Only the thinner short-jawed forceps (*far left*) is suitable for pediatric work. B: Small back-biting forceps are used to open the anterior fontanelle. C: View of an ostium after the anterior fontanelle has been removed. This opening is larger than currently used in most patients.

too large a bite anteriorly for fear of damaging the lacrimal duct. The lacrimal duct is located only a short distance from the natural ostium of the sinus (Fig. 10.44).

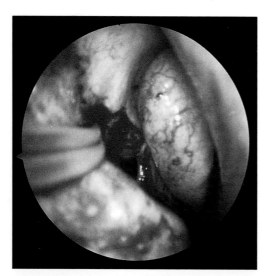

FIG. 10.44. Photo of an endoscopic dacryocystorhinoscopy. The Crawford stent can be seen exiting the lacrimal duct. A small fenestration can be seen in the anterior fontanelle just posterior to the lacrimal duct.

It is important to make sure that the opening into the maxillary sinus is connected to the natural ostium. If it is not, there will be an accumulation of secretions, which will result in persistent symptoms (Fig. 10.45). The bone along the inferior portion of the ostium is dislodged with a J curette and removed with straight- and up-biting forceps. Care is taken not to resect or traumatize the maxillary sinus mucosa. This mucosa is rolled over the inferior edge of the new ostium (Fig. 10.46A,C). If this can be performed successfully, the ostium will remain widely patent with minimal granulation tissue (Fig. 10.46B,D).

Ethmoid Bulla (Basal Lamella 2)

The pediatric ethmoid sinuses are located in a small cavity with boundaries, which if penetrated may result in significant complications. All movements within this cavity must be performed under direct visualization with deliberate calculated movements. When performing an ethmoidectomy it is necessary to gently retract the middle turbinate medially to provide adequate exposure to the cavity. As this is done, care must be taken to cause as little trauma to the mucosa of the

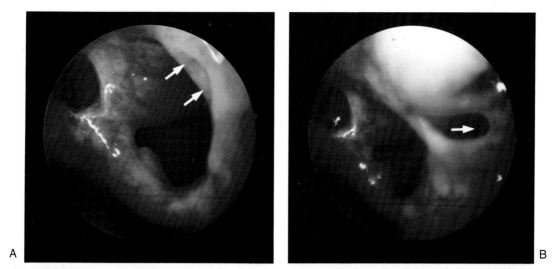

FIG. 10.45. A: Patient with persistent symptoms that consisted of secretions that look like moist mucosa and can be seen on the lateral nasal wall just anterior to the enlarged ostium (*arrow*). **B:** When the secretions are removed, the natural ostium can be identified and noted not to be connected with the enlarged ostium. Connecting the two resulted in resolution of symptoms.

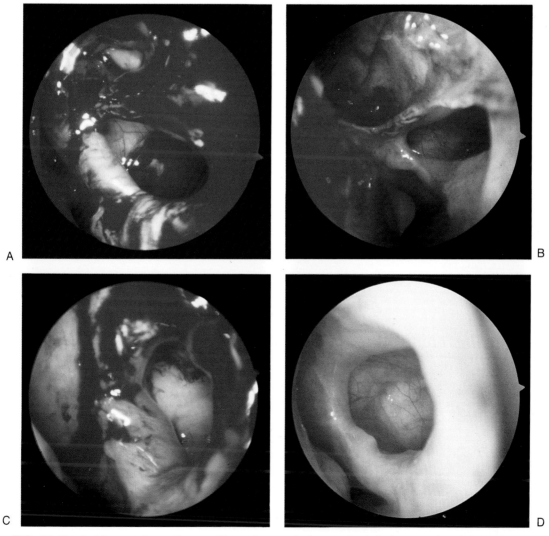

FIG. 10.46. A: Mucosa from the maxillary sinus rolled over the inferior margin of the enlarged maxillary sinus ostium. **B:** Patient A, 2 weeks postoperatively. **C:** Patient B with maxillary sinus mucosa rolled over the inferior margin. **D:** Patient B, 6 weeks postoperatively.

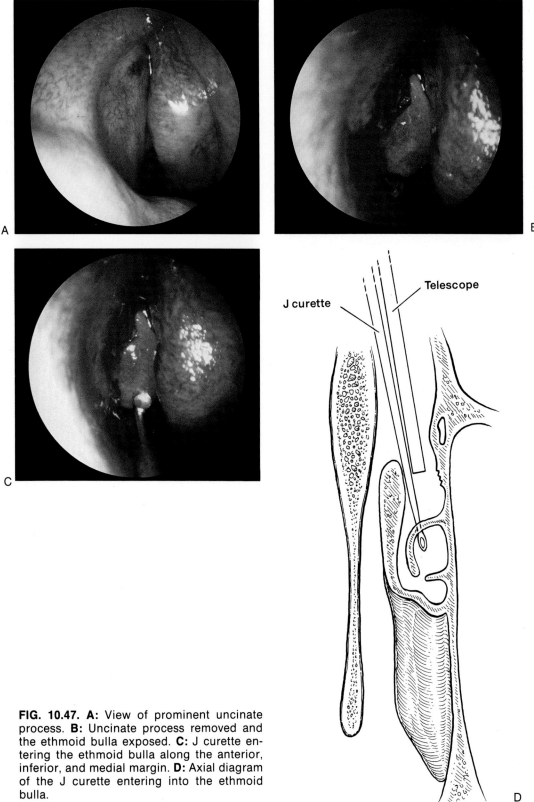

FIG. 10.47. A: View of prominent uncinate process. **B:** Uncinate process removed and the ethmoid bulla exposed. **C:** J curette entering the ethmoid bulla along the anterior, inferior, and medial margin. **D:** Axial diagram of the J curette entering into the ethmoid bulla.

J curette

Telescope

middle turbinate as possible. It has been my observation that the mucosa is traumatized most frequently with the suction.

The safest place to enter the ethmoid bulla is anterior, inferior, and medial. The bulla can be entered with minimal trauma and risk with a J curette placed in this quadrant (Fig. 10.47). The curette is forced into the bulla in a controlled manner, rotated superiorly, and withdrawn to fracture the bone outward. A 45-degree pediatric up-biting cup is then inserted into the bulla and a portion of the anterior face is removed (Fig. 10.48). The bulla is then directly examined. If there is normal mucosa within the bulla, it will not easily strip from the bone and the bulla will be seen to be clear.

If the ethmoid bulla is normal and the CT scan shows minimal disease, the procedure may be stopped at this point (Fig. 10.49). If there is diseased mucosa or purulence in the bulla, an anterior ethmoidectomy should be performed (Fig. 10.50). Once the anterior wall of the ethmoid has been removed the medial wall is removed with several small bites of the straight cups. The straight cup is advanced into the middle meatus with the inferior jaw being advanced into the space between the lateral surface of the middle turbinate and the medial surface of the ethmoid bulla (Fig. 10.51). The mobile superior jaw of the cup is advanced into the bulla. This maneuver allows the middle turbinate to be retracted and maximizes visualization of the

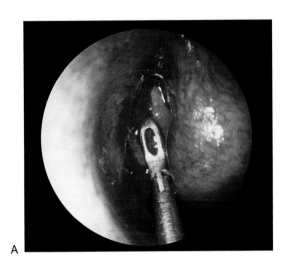

A

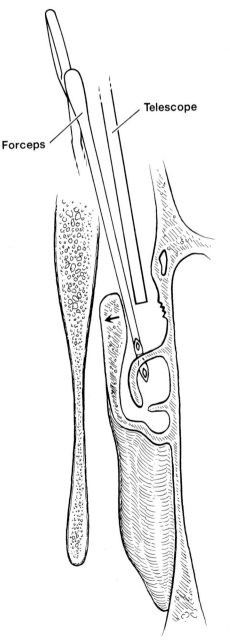

Forceps

Telescope

B

FIG. 10.48. A: A 45-degree up-biting cup removing the anterior wall of the ethmoid bulla. **B:** Axial diagram of the 45-degree cup forceps removing the anterior wall of the ethmoid bulla.

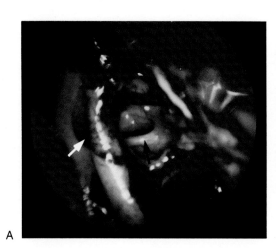 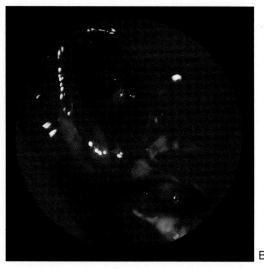

FIG. 10.49. A: Anterior wall of a normal ethmoid bulla removed. Note the widely patent posterior wall opening into the sinus lateralis (*arrow*). **B:** Another patient with a maxillary antrostomy and a normal opened ethmoid bulla.

bulla. The medial wall of the bulla will guide the surgeon to the juncture of the middle turbinate and medial wall of the ethmoid bulla or into a space behind the ethmoid bulla known as the sinus lateralis or the hiatus semilunaris superiorus (Grunwald). The sinus lateralis can extend a variable distance superiorly over the bulla and toward the roof of the ethmoid cavity. The sinus lateralis or the juncture of the middle turbinate and the bulla is the best landmark for the third and most developed basal lamella (Fig. 10.52). Posterior to this lamella are the posterior ethmoid cells. The dissection is carried superiorly, but the roof of the ethmoid bulla is not identified at this time and the frontal recess is not entered.

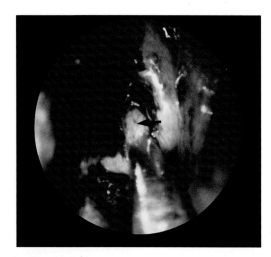

FIG. 10.50. Diseased mucosa (*arrow*) in the ethmoid bulla.

Lamina Papyracea

If an anterior ethmoidectomy is performed, the entire ethmoid bulla should be removed. To do this the lamina papyracea must be clearly identified. If the maxillary ostium has been identified or a maxillary antrostomy performed, the level of the floor of the orbit can easily be identified (Figs. 10.49B and 10.53). By using a 30-degree telescope, the mucosa can gently be removed and the lamina papyracea can clearly be identified by its smooth texture and yellow color (Fig. 10.54). This is a clear boundary that can be followed into the posterior ethmoid. Diseased mucosa should be removed superiorly up to but not into the frontal recess. If the mucosa is normal, it should be preserved (Fig. 10.55). Special care should be used when removing the mucosa at the juncture of the lamina papyracea and the floor of the orbit because this is where the bone is the thinnest and the area where orbital fat is most likely to be obtained. If the surgeon operates from the right side of the patient, the left orbit is most likely to be penetrated.

Basal Lamella and Posterior Ethmoid Cells

Identification of the third basal lamella is important because it marks the anterior border of the posterior ethmoid cells. Once the ethmoid bulla has been removed in its entirety the basal (ground) lamella will be clearly seen (Fig. 10.55B,C). Rarely is it a flat plate. It is an ill-defined bony connection between the lamina papyracea and the middle turbinate and may have deep invaginations of the sinus lateralis. The posterior eth-

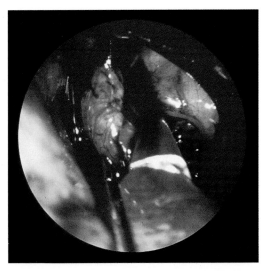

A

FIG. 10.51. A: Straight cups removing the medial wall of the ethmoid bulla. The medial wall can be used as a guide to the sinus lateralis or the basal lamella. **B:** Axial diagram of straight cups removing the medial wall of the ethmoid bulla.

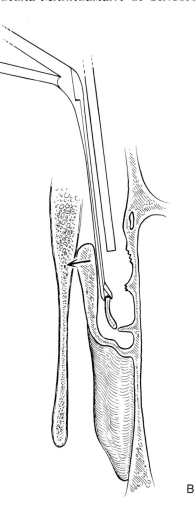

B

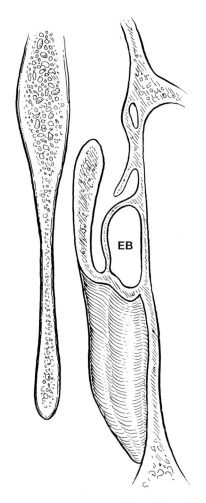

FIG. 10.52. Axial diagram of the ethmoid bulla meeting the middle turbinate and no evidence of a sinus lateralis.

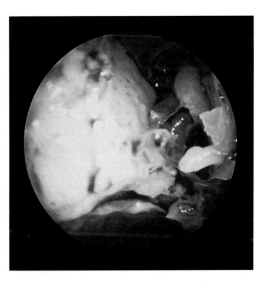

FIG. 10.53. The ostium of the maxillary sinus will help locate the floor of the orbit and the lamina papyracea. (Pediatric cadaver dissection.)

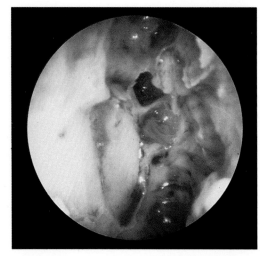

FIG. 10.54. View of the lamina papyracea with a 30-degree telescope. Note the yellow color and the smooth texture of the bone. Dissection is carried up to the region of the frontal recess. If the bone is palpated the entire lateral wall can be seen to move slightly. (Pediatric cadaver dissection.)

moid cells can also bulge anteriorly into the lumen of the anterior ethmoid. The posterior cells are much larger and the roof of the ethmoid is much easier to identify posteriorly. The ground lamella may also be identified by placing the telescope into the posterior middle meatus. The posterior middle meatus is formed by two walls of the middle turbinate: a vertical (side) and a horizontal (roof) segment (Fig. 10.56). A 2.7-mm telescope can frequently be rolled into the posterior middle meatus and the horizontal ground lamella followed anteriorly until it takes a nearly vertical course (Fig. 10.56). This marks the portion of the ground lamella that should be perforated in the safest area, which is medial and inferior (Fig. 10.57). The perforation may lead directly into the superior meatus. The middle meatus can be visualized from the medial side (Fig. 10.57D) and from the lateral side (Fig. 10.57E) of the middle turbinate. Careful observation of the medial side of the dissection (along the middle turbinate) will allow identification of the superior meatus and the precise identification of the position of the dissection.

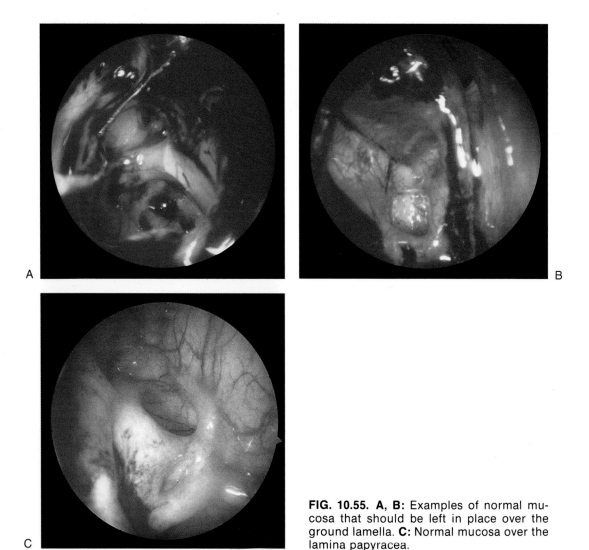

FIG. 10.55. A, B: Examples of normal mucosa that should be left in place over the ground lamella. **C:** Normal mucosa over the lamina papyracea.

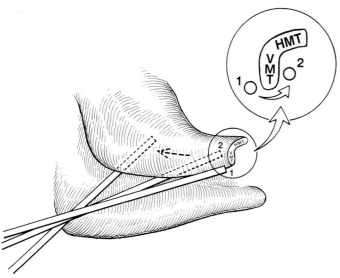

FIG. 10.56. Diagrammatic drawing of a 2.7-mm telescope being rotated into the posterior middle meatus and coming forward to identify the ground lamella. The posterior middle turbinate is composed of a vertical segment (VMT) and a horizontal segment (HMT).

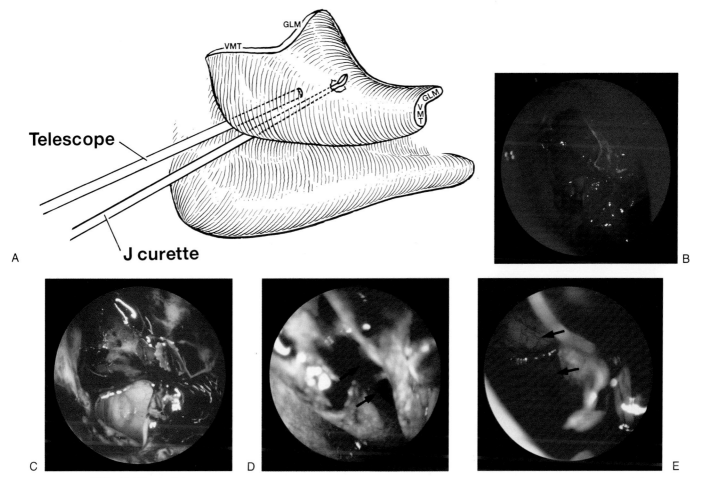

FIG. 10.57. A: Diagrammatic representation of the J curette piercing the ground lamella at the inferior medial border. **B:** The posterior ethmoid cell has been opened along the medial inferior border. **C:** A closer view of the normal posterior ethmoid cell. **D:** View of the superior meatus (*arrow*) from the medial side of the middle turbinate. **E:** View of the superior meatus (*arrow*) within the ethmoid cavity.

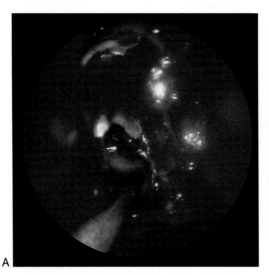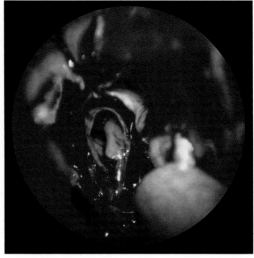

FIG. 10.58. Views of posterior ethmoid cells that have been entered and are not diseased; therefore they are left intact.

The basal lamella can be penetrated in a controlled manner with the J curette and straight cups. The mucosa from the posterior cells should be removed carefully in an attempt to leave any normal mucosa along the roof of the ethmoid. Frequently, only the bone is removed and the posterior sinus mucosa is left intact. If this occurs, grabbing the mucosa with forceps will strip the mucosa from the sinus. It is better to incise the mucosa with a myringotomy knife and look into the sinus (Fig. 10.58). The mucosa from the posterior cells should be removed carefully in an attempt to leave any normal mucosa along the roof of the ethmoid. If these cells are free of disease, the posterior cells can be left intact. As with adults, the forceps should be directed laterally along the roof to prevent penetration through the (medial) cribriform plate. The most posterior ethmoid cell, the Onodi cell, shows varying degrees of development in children (Fig. 10.59). The Onodi cell may be quite large. It is my impression that the optic nerve is somewhat more protected than in adults, but many teenagers show extensive development of the sinuses and I have seen the optic nerve in the posterior ethmoid of a 7-year-old.

Sphenoid Sinus

The sphenoid is not as frequently diseased in children and therefore is not frequently opened. Passing

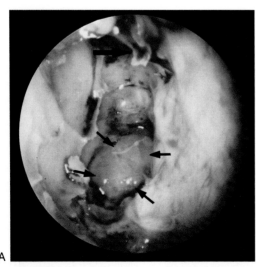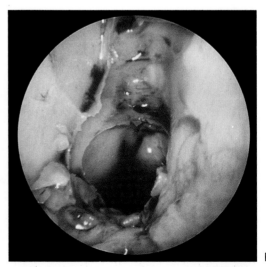

FIG. 10.59. Normal posterior ethmoid cells that can be used to identify the roof of the ethmoid cells and then to dissect forward into the anterior ethmoid cells. **A:** The wall posteriorly (*arrow*) represents the posterior-most ethmoid cell (Onodi cell) that has not been opened. Note the clearly defined roof of the ethmoid cells and the remnants of the anterior cells (*large arrow*). **B:** The Onodi cell has been opened. Note the extension of the roof posteriorly along the same plane. (Pediatric cadaver dissection.) (See Fig. 10.62 for location of sphenoid.)

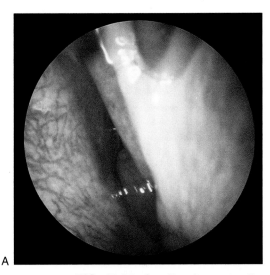
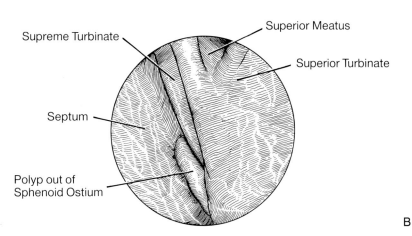

Supreme Turbinate

Superior Meatus

Superior Turbinate

Septum

Polyp out of
Sphenoid Ostium

A

B

FIG. 10.60. Small polyp extruding from the sphenoid recess in a 10-year-old patient with aspergillus infection of the right posterior ethmoid and sphenoid sinuses.

a 2.7-mm scope into the recess frequently results in trauma and edema to the mucosa and the limited space does not allow for good instrument manipulation (Fig. 10.60). It is therefore necessary to open the sphenoid through the posterior ethmoid cells.

On the coronal CT scan the sphenoid is located in a position directly behind the posterior ethmoid with the roof usually lower than the ethmoid. On visualization through the endoscope, the sphenoid is located much lower and more medially than one would anticipate from the CT scan. The reasons for this are twofold. First, the endoscopes have a wide angle of view, and the amount of distortion is not readily appreciated by the surgeon (Fig. 10.61). Second, the coronal CT scan is oriented in a different plane than the 30 to 40 degrees off-axis that the surgeon is operating in. This

results in the appearance of the sphenoid being much lower than should be anticipated by the coronal CT scan (Fig. 10.62).

I have found it easiest to enter the sphenoid through the posterior ethmoid with a J curette and straight forceps. One should be very cautious along the lateral and superior wall of the sphenoid and posterior ethmoid sinus. It is difficult to use instruments in the sphenoid sinus of children because of limited space. If one is uncertain of the sphenoid, the suspected site can first be aspirated with a needle or the position of the sphenoid can be checked through the natural ostium. The level of the roof can be located by finding the natural ostium of the sphenoid through the sphenoid recess.

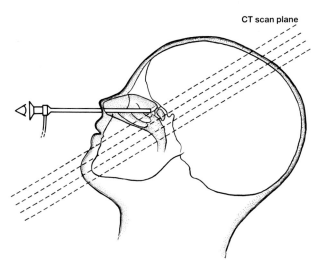

CT scan plane

FIG. 10.61. Diagram of the orientation of the CT scans and the surgeon's view through the telescope.

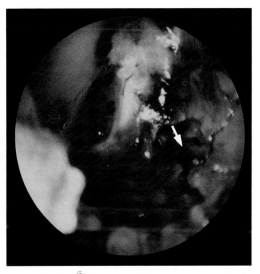

FIG. 10.62. Pediatric cadaver dissection of posterior ethmoid cells with a sucker (*arrow*) protruding through the natural ostium into the posterior ethmoid cells.

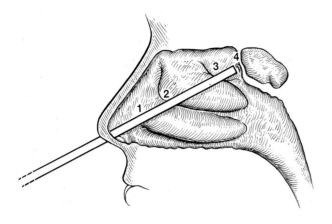

FIG. 10.63. Diagram showing a reliable route to the sphenoid ostium: (1) view at the root of the inferior turbinate; (2) view at the inferior third of the middle turbinate; (3) view at the inferior third of the superior turbinate; (4) view of the sphenoid recess with a polyp extruding from the sphenoid ostium.

The best landmarks to the sphenoid recess are noted in Fig. 10.63. A line along the root of the inferior turbinate and the lower third of the middle and superior turbinates will guide the surgeon to the sphenoid ostium (Fig. 10.60). Figure 10.64 details the surgical dissection in a 10-year-old child with posterior ethmoid and sphenoid opacification. The CT scans clearly delineate the extent of the disease (Fig. 10.64).

Frontal Recess and Agger Nasi Cells

Once the level of the roof of the ethmoid has been identified in the posterior cells, the plane of the roof can be followed into the anterior ethmoid cells (Fig. 10.65). If the mucosa along the roof is normal, every effort should be made to leave it intact. The appropriate management of the developing frontal recess and frontal sinus is not clear. We unfortunately have no prospective or retrospective data on effects of surgery in this area in children. It therefore would seem prudent to be very conservative in the frontal recess until more is known about development with surgery. I do not invade the frontal recess if the mucosa appears normal and free of disease (Fig. 10.66). The seeker is an ideal instrument to gently move mucosa and small fragments of bone when inspecting the frontal recess. When the recess is opened, every effort is made to leave the normal mucosa intact (Figs. 10.67 and 10.68). When there is extensive disease, the mucosa will sometimes strip out in one piece, even when taking small bites. When this occurs it is appropriate to open the area as much as possible. The agger nasi cells are present in most children and can be opened with a 90-degree forceps or the 90-degree J curette. As long as the instruments are not forced superiorly, this can be performed safely. These cells may be hard to visualize but should be removed if the frontal recess is to be explored.

Postoperative Care

The postoperative care for the pediatric sinus endoscopy patient is modified from that used in adults because of poor patient cooperation. Postoperatively, even anterior rhinoscopy cannot be performed in some patients. Any postoperative cleaning must therefore be performed under general anesthesia except in the most cooperative child. We initially used Silastic, reinforced 0.02 in. thick, to hold the middle meatus open. It was our impression, however, that this produced excessive granulation tissue within the ethmoid cavity (Fig. 10.69). Because of this excessive granulation tissue, we have abandoned this method of treatment.

We then started using Gelfilm (Upjohn, Kalamazoo, MI), which was moistened for 15 s in normal saline, then rolled and placed in the middle meatus (Fig. 10.70). It is important to emphasize that Gelfilm and *NOT Gelfoam* is placed in the middle meatus. Surgeons who have used Gelfoam report a higher incidence of scarring in the meatus. The surgeon must be assured that the Gelfilm has been placed lateral to the middle turbinate. If placed medially, it will force the meatus closed and virtually assure postoperative scarring.

The posterior portion of the Gelfilm should be against the basal lamella or into the posterior ethmoid cavity to prevent the child from blowing the stent out (Fig. 10.71). If the stents are appropriately placed in the middle meatus, the child will be able to breath through the nose with minimal problems. As crusting and purulence develop around the Gelfilm, the airway patency decreases.

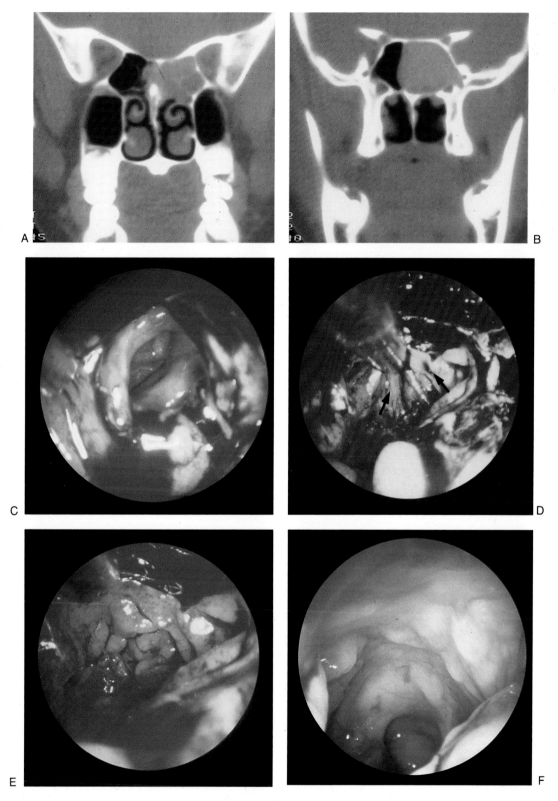

FIG. 10.64. This 10-year-old who presented with recurrent headaches. **A, B:** Coronal CT scans of the patient show unilateral posterior ethmoid and sphenoid sinus disease. **C:** Opening into the anterior-most posterior ethmoid cells. Note the normal mucosa. **D:** Sphenoid sinus filled with very thick tenacious secretions (*arrow*). **E:** Sphenoid sinus after the secretions had been removed in their entirety. **F:** Sphenoid sinus 2 weeks postoperatively.

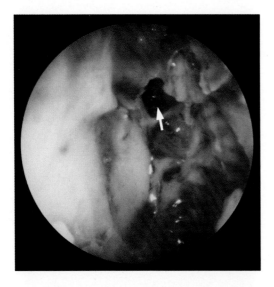

FIG. 10.65. Pediatric cadaver dissection with the roof of the ethmoid defined posteriorly. The dissection is progressing anteriorly into the anterior ethmoid cells and frontal recess (*arrow*).

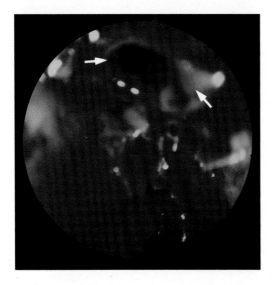

FIG. 10.66. The diseased mucosa has gently been removed, leaving relatively normal mucosa (*arrow*) in the area of the frontal recess.

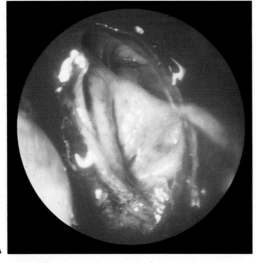
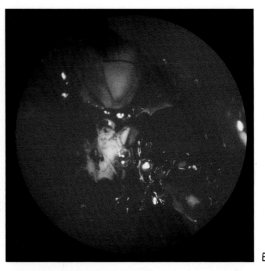

A   B

FIG. 10.67. View of normal mucosa leading into the widened frontal recesses of two patients. Note that no effort is made to remove this normal mucosa.

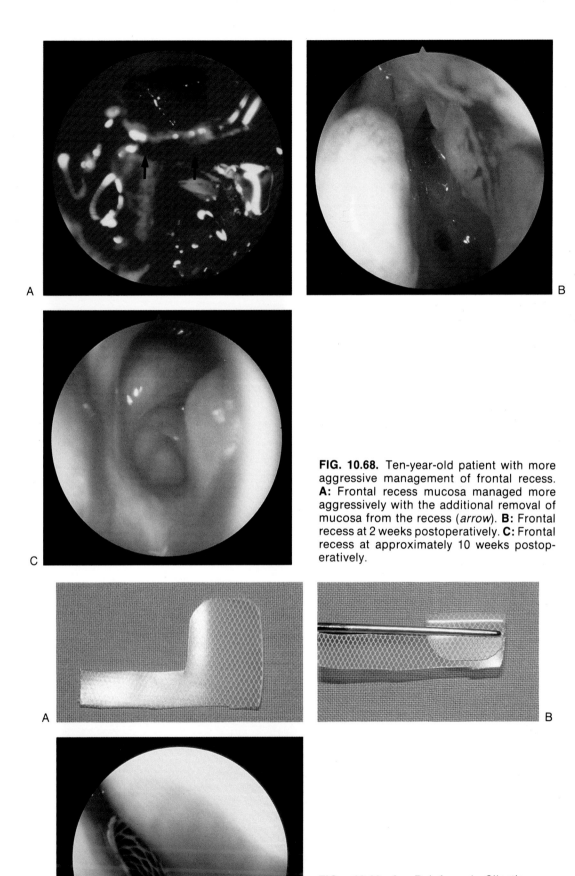

FIG. 10.68. Ten-year-old patient with more aggressive management of frontal recess. **A:** Frontal recess mucosa managed more aggressively with the additional removal of mucosa from the recess (*arrow*). **B:** Frontal recess at 2 weeks postoperatively. **C:** Frontal recess at approximately 10 weeks postoperatively.

FIG. 10.69. A: Reinforced Silastic sheeting cut to extend along the septum and rolled into the ethmoid cavity. **B:** Silastic positioned for insertion. **C:** Silastic stent in the middle meatus holding the lateral wall of the nose and middle turbinate apart. **Note: Silastic is now rarely used in our practice.**

113

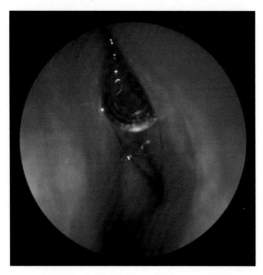

FIG. 10.70. Gelfilm rolled and placed into the middle meatus.

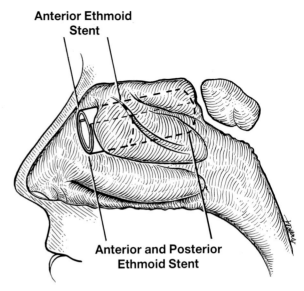

Anterior Ethmoid
Stent

Anterior and Posterior
Ethmoid Stent

FIG. 10.71. Diagram of the length and position of Gelfilm for an anterior and anterior–posterior ethmoidectomy.

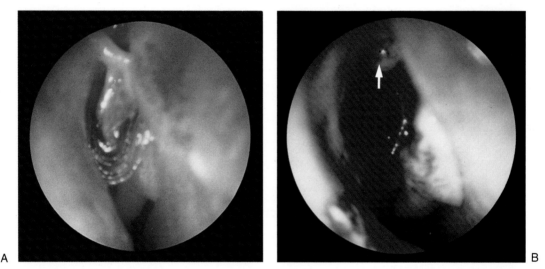

A

B

FIG. 10.72. A: Rolled Gelfilm in place for 2 weeks. **B:** Ethmoid cavity after removing the Gelfilm roll. Note the near total occlusion of the frontal recess with granulation tissue (*arrow*).

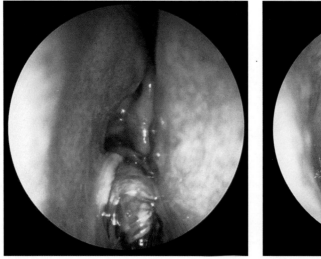

A

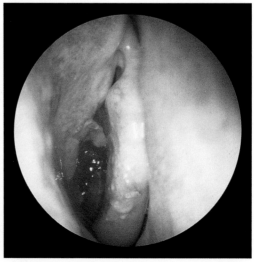

B

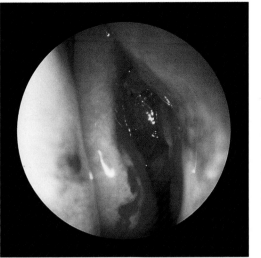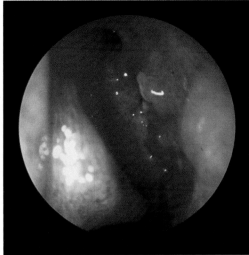

FIG. 10.74. Two patients 2 weeks after surgery with the Gelfilm roll removed.

Experience has taught us that the Gelfilm should be removed under a general anesthetic at approximately 2 weeks postoperatively. When removed, a fair amount of purulence will be seen around the Gelfilm (Figs. 10.72A and 10.73A). The Gelfilm is best removed with an alligator forceps, by gently grasping it inferiorly and rocking the stent up and down until it is loose enough to be removed. The Gelfilm is fragile and easily fragments if it is grasped too firmly.

A variable amount of granulation tissue accumulates in the area of the frontal recess and the maxillary an-

trostomy (Figs. 10.72B, 10.73B, and 10.74A,B). If the mucosa from the maxillary sinus can be rolled over the inferior edge, there will be little granulation tissue in the ostium (Fig. 10.46). The granulation tissue around the frontal recess and maxillary ostium should be gently removed, but no effort is made to clean all the granulation tissue in the rest of the cavity. A half to a full roll of Gelfilm is placed back in the cavity (Fig. 10.75).

The patient is kept on full-dose antibiotics until the stent falls out or has absorbed (usually within 2 to 3

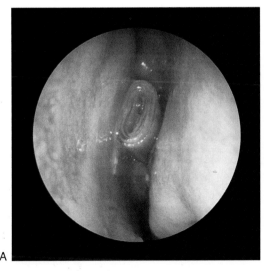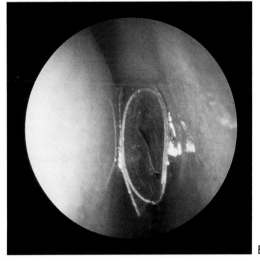

A   B

FIG. 10.75. A: Full Gelfilm roll placed back in the ethmoid cavity. **B:** Half of Gelfilm roll placed back into the cavity.

FIG. 10.73. A: Rolled Gelfilm in place for 2 weeks. Note that the roll has slipped inferiorly and has not remained at the root of the middle turbinate. **B:** Ethmoid cavity after removing the Gelfilm roll.

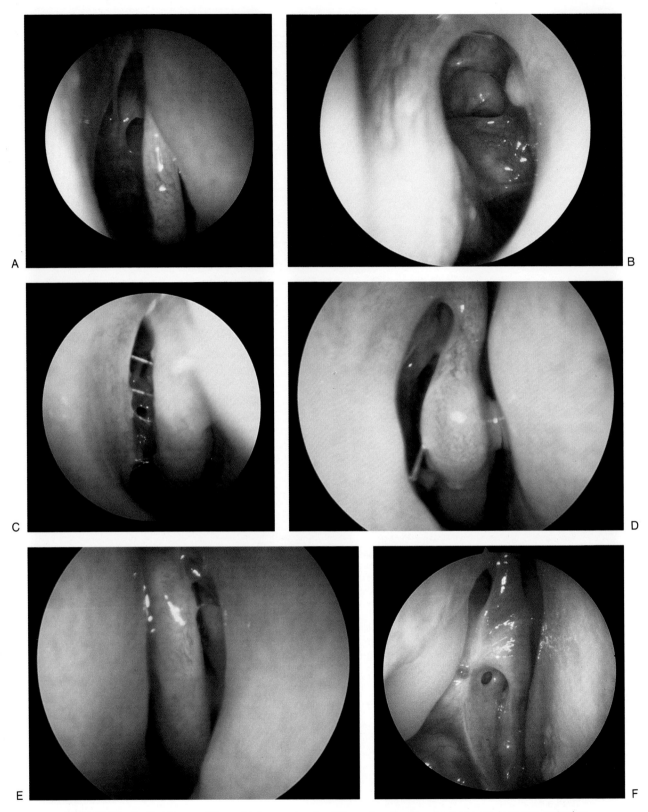

FIG. 10.76. A–H: Views of the middle meatus in different patients who have undergone anterior ethmoidectomy. The ground lamella and the lack of scarring between the middle turbinate and lateral wall of the nose are clearly demonstrated. **C, D:** Mucus and not scarring are noted between the middle turbinate and lateral wall. Part (**C**) shows some residual uncinate process that was incompletely removed at the time of surgery but has not complicated the postoperative result. **F:** View taken with a 30-degree telescope and looking at the frontal recess. **H:** View of small cavities in a child who had an anterior ethmoidectomy. The telescope is positioned just beyond the middle turbinate. Note the clearly demonstrated ground lamella without evidence of scarring.

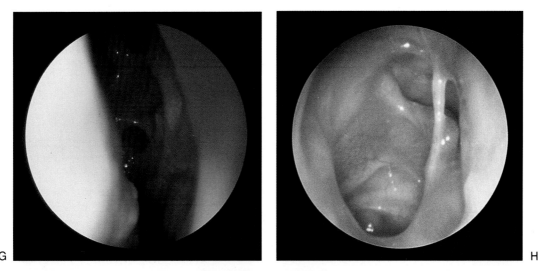

FIG. 10.76. (*Continued*)

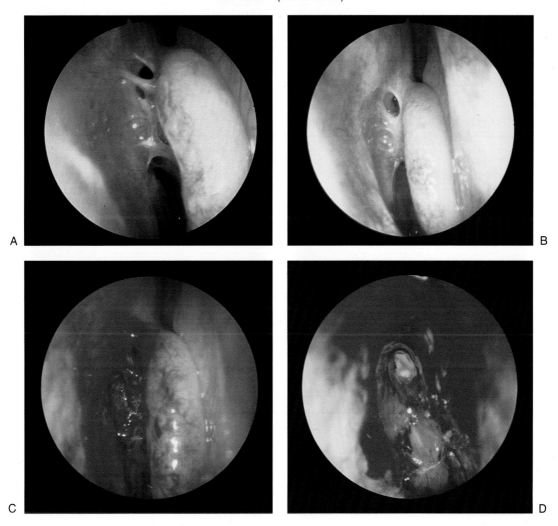

FIG. 10.77. A: Scarring in the superior middle meatus after an ethmoidectomy in an adolescent patient with cystic fibrosis. Gelfilm stent was not placed because of the size of the cavity and the feeling that the cavity could be adequately cleaned postoperatively. **B:** Lesser degree of scarring after revision of the same patient in the same area as Fig. 10.77A. **C:** Patient continued to complain of right frontal headaches; therefore, another revision ethmoidectomy was undertaken. This figure depicts the scar being removed. **D:** The frontal recess revealed typical thick secretions of a patient with cystic fibrosis in frontal recess.

weeks). Prophylactic antibiotics are used until the cavity is free of crusting. Prospective studies have *not* been performed to ascertain the necessity of antibiotics throughout the entire postoperative period or if the second look, at 2 weeks, is necessary.

Scarring using this method has been virtually nonexistent (Figs. 10.46D, 10.65E, 10.68C, 10.76A–D, and 10.78A). When we have deviated from this routine, we have had problems with scarring (Fig. 10.77).

On occasion a scar will form between the middle turbinate and lateral wall of the nose. This scar may be small (Fig. 10.78A) or substantial and cause significant obstruction. This problem can be prevented if the Gelfilm is extended beyond the ethmoid cavity and between the middle turbinate and lateral wall of the nose (Fig. 10.78B,C).

The success of the surgical intervention is best assessed by resolution of the patient's symptoms. A follow-up CT scan, particularly if sedation is required, seems unwarranted if the patient is asymptomatic. If the patient is symptomatic and must continue antibiotic therapy to remain clear, then a repeat CT scan

would seem warranted. Figure 10.79A is the preoperative CT scan of a 4-year-old patient with persistent symptoms of chronic sinusitis. He underwent endoscopic sinus surgery and had intermittent symptoms, so a repeat CT scan was performed; the results are shown in Fig. 10.79B. Good resolution of the maxillary and ethmoid sinus disease can be seen. There was a small amount of isolated right agger nasi cell disease (Fig. 10.79C) that was observed. Figure 10.80 depicts a child with symptoms 1 month after an anterior ethmoidectomy. The coronal CT scan was repeated during a time when a prospective study was being performed to assess the accuracy of the plain films; therefore a set of plain films was also obtained (Fig. 10.80A). Note the opacified right maxillary sinus and thickened mucosa of the left maxillary sinus. The CT scan (Fig. 10.80B) revealed widely patent maxillary antrostomies and mucosal thickening of the right maxillary sinus and the roof of the left maxillary sinus. The posterior ethmoid cells are free of disease. Mucous membrane thickening of the maxillary sinus consistently causes opacification of the sinus on plain films.

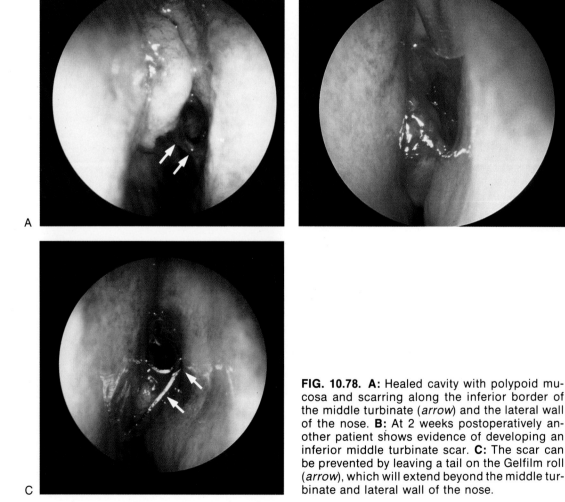

FIG. 10.78. A: Healed cavity with polypoid mucosa and scarring along the inferior border of the middle turbinate (*arrow*) and the lateral wall of the nose. **B:** At 2 weeks postoperatively another patient shows evidence of developing an inferior middle turbinate scar. **C:** The scar can be prevented by leaving a tail on the Gelfilm roll (*arrow*), which will extend beyond the middle turbinate and lateral wall of the nose.

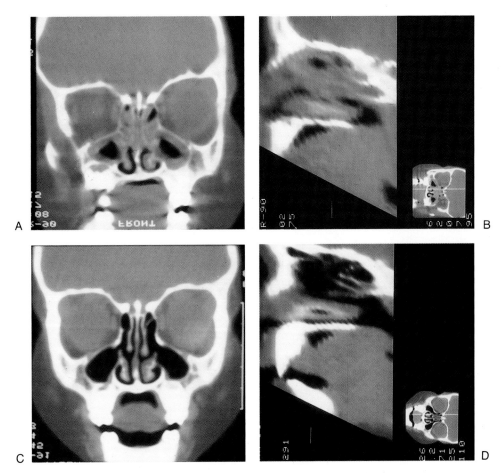

FIG. 10.79. **A, B:** Coronal and sagittal reconstruction of a patient with symptoms of ethmoid disease significant enough to warrant endoscopic ethmoidectomy. **C, D:** Coronal and sagittal reconstruction of the postoperative CT scans showing good resolution of disease.

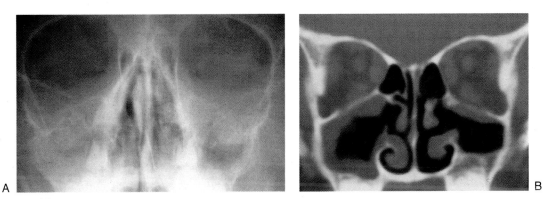

FIG. 10.80. **A:** Plain film of postoperative patient. Note the opacification of the right maxillary sinus and the mucous membrane thickening of the left maxillary sinus. Also note that it is difficult to make any assessment of the ethmoid sinuses. **B:** Coronal CT scan reveals mucous membrane thickening of the right maxillary sinus and only slight thickening of the mucous membrane over the roof of the left maxillary sinus.

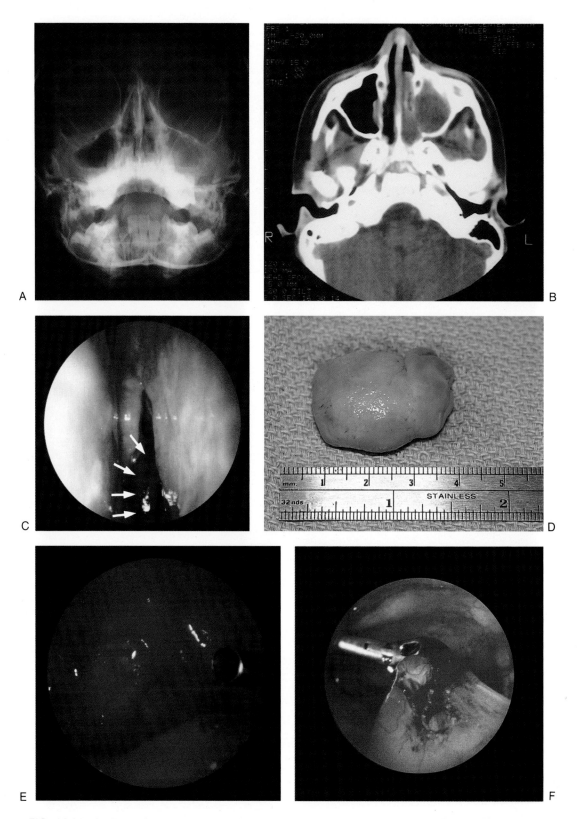

FIG. 10.81. A: Plain films of patient with left choanal polyp. **B:** Axial CT scan of the choanal polyp. Note the opacification of the left maxillary sinus and nasal airway. **C:** Anterior rhinoscopy reveals a polyp (*arrow*) extruding from the inferior middle meatus. **D:** Choanal polyp that had to be delivered through the mouth. **E:** Trocar placed through the canine fossa and viewed with a 70-degree telescope. **F:** Garaff forceps removing residual choanal polyp from the floor and lateral wall of the maxillary sinus. The forceps is introduced through the ostium of the maxillary sinus and visualized through the canine fossa with a 0-degree telescope.

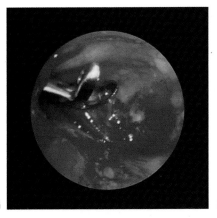 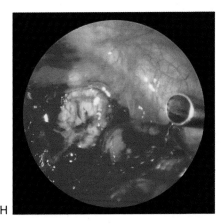 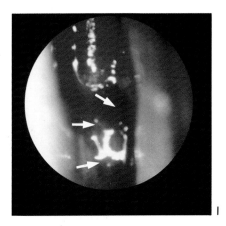

G H I

FIG. 10.81. (*Continued*) **G:** The 45-degree forceps can be used to remove residual mucosa. **H:** The removed mucosa of the lateral wall and floor of the maxillary sinus is clearly visualized through a 70-degree telescope. Note the trocar remaining in place through the canine fossa. **I:** Recurrence of the choanal polyp (*arrow*).

SPECIAL SURGICAL PROCEDURES

Choanal Polyps

Choanal polyps can be difficult to manage. They arise from the maxillary sinus and extend into the nasal cavity. On occasion they are large enough to completely obstruct the nasopharynx. Plain films and coronal CT scans will reveal opacification of the maxillary sinus and nasal airway (Fig. 10.81A,B). On examination of the nasal airway a large polypoid mass can be seen extruding from the inferior middle meatus (Fig. 10.81C). The polyp is frequently large enough that it must be delivered through the mouth (Fig. 10.81D). The polyp can arise from the anterior, medial, or lateral wall or the roof or floor of the maxillary sinus. All the mucosa from the site of origin of the cyst must be removed. This can be difficult to impossible to perform endoscopically. Frequently, the telescope will have to be placed into the maxillary sinus through the canine fossa to maximize visualization of the site of origin (Fig. 10.81E). The telescope can be used to guide instruments introduced through the enlarged ostium of the maxillary sinus (Fig. 10.81F,G). The Garaff forceps can be used to remove polypoid mucosa from the lateral wall and floor of the maxillary sinus (Fig. 10.81F). The anterior wall is difficult to reach with forceps (Fig. 10.81G). A 70-degree telescope can be used to examine the lateral and lateral–anterior wall of the maxillary sinus (Fig. 10.81H). The incidence of recurrence is rather high and the cyst looks much the same as the primary lesion (Fig. 10.81I). It may be necessary to perform a Caldwell–Luc procedure through a limited anterior approach to remove all mucosa from the anterior or medial walls.

Dacryocystorhinostomy

The intranasal approach to the lacrimal duct is greatly facilitated with endoscopic telescopes and techniques. Perhaps the single most significant advance is the use of the light pipe (Storz, St. Louis, MO) (Fig. 10.82A) to cannulate the duct. The advantage is that the lacrimal duct can be illuminated from within the duct and clearly identified in the nose through transillumination (Fig. 10.82B). If the transilluminated light is difficult to identify, the telescope light can be decreased to improve visualization (Fig. 10.82C). Vasoconstrictors (oxymetazoline) are placed on the mucosa and 1:100,000 epinephrine is injected into the mucosa. An incision is then placed over the area of illumination and the bone identified (Fig. 10.82D). Once the bone is exposed a J curette is used to remove the bone and a myringotomy knife is used to incise the duct. The Crawford stents are guided through the lacrimal ducts and then pulled out through the nose under endoscopic visualization (Fig. 10.44).

SURGICAL COMPLICATIONS

The surgical complications of pediatric disease have so far been few; I am personally unaware of any complications in children. The procedure, however, can be expected to have potential complications similar to those in adult surgery. Some surgeons suggest that the risk of complications may even be higher in children because of the smaller anatomical spaces in which one must work. Stankiewicz (66) showed the importance of acquiring experience in endoscopic techniques through appropriate didactic training and multiple ca-

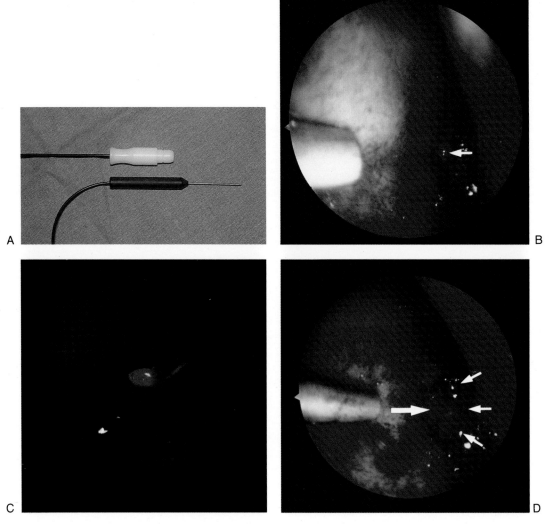

FIG. 10.82. A: Photo of retinal probe. **B:** View of the lateral wall with the retinal probe causing transillumination of the lacrimal duct (*arrow*). **C:** View of the transilluminate light from the duct with the light of the telescope turned off. **D:** Incision of the mucosa over the lacrimal duct (*small arrow*) and the bone overlying the duct exposed (*large arrow*).

daver dissections and demonstrated that experience decreases the complication rate (67). An accurate knowledge of the anatomy and prudent judgment will decrease risks to an acceptable level.

Hemorrhage itself can be considered a complication. Stankiewicz (66) noted that 5 of 90 patients had significant bleeding at the time of surgery, but he noted no subsequent episodes of major bleeding (67). It has been our experience in over 300 patients that significant hemorrhage is rare in the pediatric population. We have on three occasions aborted the procedure because of bleeding that (less than 100 cc) resulted in persistent poor visualization. Two of the patients were part of a protocol evaluating phenylephrine as a vasoconstrictor.

Most bleeding is capillary in nature, but even small amounts of bleeding can be a problem in endoscopic sinus surgery. In such cases it is best to stop the procedure and pack the cavity with neuropledgets saturated with a vasoconstrictor; we prefer 0.05% oxymetazoline. If the bleeding persists, an effective way to control it is to make a slurry of Avitene (Medchem Products, Woburn, MA) and place it into a syringe. The slurry is then injected into the cavity and a neuropledget is placed for 5 to 10 min. I have found this to be a very effective method of controlling intraoperative bleeding. Most of the Avitene should be removed after the neuropledget has been removed to prevent excessive scarring postoperatively. Significant complications are most frequently secondary to excessive bleeding, poor visualization, and poor judgment.

The complications can be classified in two broad categories: orbital and intracranial.

Orbital Complications

Orbital complications can occur in the form of (a) blindness secondary to direct injury to the optic nerve or secondary to retrobulbar hemorrhage, (b) diplopia secondary to trauma to the orbital muscles or secondary fibrosis, and (c) epiphora secondary to trauma to the lacrimal duct. The best prevention of these complications is a thorough knowledge of the anatomy in general and specifically of any congenital anomalies in the patient. Congenital dehiscences are sometimes noted in the wall of the orbit, in the lamina papyracea, or over the posterior ethmoid cells. If these are recognized preoperatively, the chance of trauma is reduced.

Blindness secondary to direct optic nerve injury is rare but has occurred (68,69). Trauma is most likely to occur in the sphenoid or Onodi (the posterior-most ethmoid cell) in adults. These cells are less developed in children and therefore perhaps are less likely to be traumatized. An isolated injury to the optic nerve without associated trauma to the other orbital contents would be unlikely (69).

The afferent pupillary defect consists of a diminished amplitude of the pupillary light reaction, a lengthened latent period, and pupillary dilation with continuous light stimulation (69) (Fig. 11.7). This is known as Marcus Gunn's syndrome and may be the first indication of optic nerve injury. A dilated pupil with the presence of vision and pupillary reflexes probably is secondary to local anesthesia and usually resolves. Deep general anesthesia will alter the pupillary response and may confuse the examination. It is wise to periodically check the pupil during and at the end of the surgical procedure. As a general rule, direct trauma to the optic nerve is irreversible.

Blindness may also occur secondary to retrobulbar or orbital hemorrhage. Orbital hemorrhage is the most frequently reported ophthalmic complication of sinus surgery (66,70,71). Its hallmarks are lid edema, lid ecchymosis, chemosis, mydriasis, and proptosis (69). It is important that the eye is not covered or sewn shut during the procedure so that the surgeon and the assistants will be able to detect the earliest changes. Subtle eye movements or movements of the lids will be the earliest manifestations of a breach of the lamina papyracea. Another early consequence of penetration of the lamina papyracea is subconjunctival hemorrhage from the orbital fat, a lacerated medial rectus muscle, or blood from the sinus cavity itself (68). More significant bleeding can occur if the anterior or posterior ethmoid arteries are transected and bleed into the orbit. If the orbital fat is thought to be exposed, the area should be carefully examined. Pressure on the orbit will cause the fat to herniate into the ethmoid cavity and this is a very useful diagnostic tool. Bleeding may occur without interruption of the lamina papyracea.

Visual loss during a retrobulbar hemorrhage is probably secondary to compromise of the central retinal artery flow (72–74) and posterior ciliary artery flow, which supply the blood to the optic nerve (74,75). There is a sense of urgency about the relief of pressure from the developing hematoma, because recovery of vision is unlikely if retinal ischemia persists for more than 100 min (76). Orbital hemorrhage may also cause paresis of the extrinsic ocular muscles, which will resolve with time (69,77). For a more extensive discussion of the causes of visual loss, see the chapter by Lusk et al.

Prevention of orbital bleeding is the key to preventing the complication. A thorough history should be obtained about bleeding disorders and medications such as aspirin or aspirin-containing products, which may result in bleeding. It may be appropriate to obtain screening clotting studies on all patients (69). Hypertension is also a factor in orbital hematoma. If the patient has had a previous procedure, it is imperative to obtain another coronal CT scan to look for anatomical abnormalities that would increase the chance of an orbital complication. Intraoperatively, the surgeon may use palpation of the orbit with observation of the lateral wall of the cavity to pick up dehiscence of the lamina papyracea.

In the pediatric population, the operation can be performed only under general anesthesia. The surgeon therefore must be particularly vigilant while performing the surgery. Local anesthetic can be used in addition, which will give better control of the bleeding. The patient's head should be elevated, and the surgeon should be operating from a sitting position. The eyes should be protected with a lubricating agent but not taped so that movement can easily be seen. If visualization is not satisfactory or if the surgeon is unsure of the position within the ethmoid cavity, it is prudent to terminate the procedure. If complications such as lid edema, ecchymosis, proptosis, or pupillary changes are noted, the procedure must be terminated to decrease risk of further injury and one should consider further tests and ophthalmology evaluation. A key factor in preventing injury is to know the precise anatomy of the patient. This can best be accomplished by identifying all structures and performing the procedure in an organized and methodical manner. Freedman and Kern (70) noted an increase in the number of complications on the right side, therefore Stankiewicz (69) recommended operating on this side first. It has been our experience that the periorbital area is exposed with equal frequency on the left.

A last predisposing factor for orbital complications is the use of packing. Packing is rarely if ever needed. If there is persistent bleeding, it is easy to control with

Avitene and a short duration of packing, which is removed before awakening the patient. If excessive packing is used with a dehiscence in the orbit, pressure can cause hemodynamic compromise of the retina (69).

If blindness or another orbital complication is suspected, the treatment should be directed toward a retrobulbar hematoma. The ophthalmologist should be consulted immediately, but the otolaryngologist should begin management of the problem immediately.

Most ophthalmologists will treat the patient conservatively, and the initial management will be medical (69). Orbital decompression is used when medical management is unsuccessful. Monitoring with a Schiotz tonometer should be performed every 5 min to ensure that the pressure is decreasing. One of the initial maneuvers used is eye massage to redistribute intraocular and extraocular fluid. This maneuver can be used after first seeing orbital fat and will reduce the risk of blood accumulation and causing orbital pressure (69). Orbital massage is contraindicated in patients who have had previous eye surgery.

Acetazolamide lowers the intraocular pressure by decreasing the aqueous humor. The initial dose is 5 to 10 mg/kg/dose intravenously and can be repeated in 2 to 4 h. Mannitol given intravenously works faster than acetazolamide and reduces the intraocular pressure in 30 to 60 min. The dose is 1 to 2 g/kg and is infused as a 20% infusion (Osmitrol) and is infused over 30 to 60 min (69).

Steroids in the megadose range of 1 to 1.5 mg/kg of Decadron as a loading dose and then 0.5 mg/kg every 6 h has been recommended for blindness following facial trauma (78).

A lateral canthotomy has been recommended (68,69) to acutely decompress the orbit. A straight hemostat is used to crush the lateral canthus and soft tissues to the orbital rim. A knife or scissors is then used to transect along the lateral canthus. This procedure is usually recommended before performing medial decompression. Decompression of the orbit into the ethmoid cavity through an external incision is probably the fastest and most effective way of decompressing the orbit. The periorbit should be incised if there is evidence of surgical trauma (68,69).

Intracranial Complications

The other major complication that can occur is a CSF leak. Fortunately, this is relatively rare (67,69). The cause is usually penetration of the fovea ethmoidalis. A thorough knowledge of the anatomy is crucial to prevent this complication. A most important principle is to stay lateral to the middle turbinate. There are no standard measurements for the height, width, or length of the ethmoid cavity in pediatric patients. Distance to the anterior and posterior walls of the sphenoid sinus is not standardized in children. The dissection therefore must be meticulous by using small bits, taking care not to penetrate the roof of the ethmoid cavity.

REFERENCES

1. Birrell JF. Chronic maxillary sinusitis in children. *Arch Dis Child* 1952;27:1–9.
2. McAlister WH, Lusk RP, Muntz HR. Comparison of plain radiographs and coronal CT scans in infants and children with recurrent sinusitis. *Am J Roentgenol* 1989;153:1259–1264.
3. Preston HG. Maxillary sinusitis in children, its relation to coryza, tonsillectomy and adenoidectomy. *Va Med Mon* 1955;82:229–232.
4. Wilson TG. Surgical anatomy of ENT in the newborn. *J Laryngol Otol* 1955;69:229.
5. Shone GR. Maxillary sinus aspiration in children. What are the indications? *J Laryngol Otol* 1987;101:461–464.
6. Clark WD, Bailey BJ. Sinusitis in children. *Tex Med* 1983;79:44–47.
7. Paul D. Sinus infection and adenotonsillitis in pediatric patients. *Laryngoscope* 1981;91:997–1000.
8. Merck W. Relationship between adenoidal enlargement and maxillary sinusitis. *HNO* 1974;6:198–199.
9. Nickman NJ. Sinusitis, otitis and adenotonsillitis in children: a retrospective study. *Laryngoscope* 1978;88:117–121.
10. Mollison WM, Kendall NE. Frequency of antral infection in children. *Guy's Hosp Rep* 1922;72:225–228.
11. Crooks J, Signy AG. Accessory nasal sinusitis in childhood. *Arch Dis Child* 1936;11:281–306.
12. Gerrie J. Sinusitis in children. *Br Med J* 1939;2:363–364.
13. Carmack JW. Sinusitis in children. *Ann Otol Rhinol Laryngol* 1931;40:515–521.
14. Stevenson RS. The treatment of subacute maxillary sinusitis especially in children. *Proc R Soc Med* 1947;40:854–858.
15. Dean LW. Paranasal sinus disease in infants and young children. *JAMA* 1925;85:317–321.
16. Cleminson FJ. Nasal sinusitis in children. *J Laryngol Otol* 1921;36:505–513.
17. Walker FM. Tonsillectomy and adenoidectomy: unsatisfactory results due to chronic maxillary sinusitis. *Br Med J* 1947;II:908–910.
18. Griffiths I. Functions of tonsils and their relations to aetiology and treatment of nasal catarrh. *Lancet* 1937;2:723–729.
19. Hoshaw TC, Nickman NJ. Sinusitis and otitis in children. *Arch Otolaryngol* 1974;100:194–195.
20. Fujita A, Takahashi H, Honjo I. Etiological role of adenoids upon otitis media with effusion. *Acta Otolaryngol [Suppl] (Stockh)* 1988;454:210–213.
21. Maresh MM, Washburn AH. Paranasal sinuses from birth to late adolescence. *Am J Dis Child* 1940;60:841–861.
22. Stammberger H. Nasal and paranasal sinus endoscopy. A diagnostic and surgical approach to recurrent sinusitis. *Endoscopy* 1986;18:213–218.
23. Stammberger H. Endoscopic endonasal surgery—concepts in treatment of recurring rhinosinusitis. Part II. Surgical technique. *Otolaryngol Head Neck Surg* 1986;94:147–156.
24. Stammberger H. Endoscopic endonasal surgery—concepts in treatment of recurring rhinosinusitis. Part I. Anatomic and pathophysiologic considerations. *Otolaryngol Head Neck Surg* 1986;94:143–147.
25. Kennedy DW, Zinreich SJ, Rosenbaum AE, Johns ME. Functional endoscopic sinus surgery. Theory and diagnostic evaluation. *Arch Otolaryngol* 1985;111:576–582.
26. Ritter FN. A clinical and anatomical study of the various techniques of irrigation of the maxillary sinus. *Laryngoscope* 1977;87:215–223.
27. Kennedy DW, Zinreich SJ, Shaalan H, Kuhn F, Naclerio R, Loch E. Endoscopic middle meatal antrostomy: theory, technique, and patency. *Laryngoscope* 1987;97:1–9.

28. Van Alyea OE. *Nasal sinus and anatomical and clinical considerations.* Baltimore: Williams & Wilkins, 1942.
29. Myerson MC. The natural orifice of the maxillary sinus. *Arch Otolaryngol* 1932;15:80–91.
30. Lund VJ. Inferior meatal antrostomy. Fundamental considerations of design and function. *J Laryngol Otol [Suppl]* 1988;15:1–18.
31. Krause H. Instrumente rach Dr. Krause. *Monatsschr Ohrenheilkunde* 1887;21:70.
32. Mikulicz J. Zur operativen Behandlung das Kempyens der Highmorshohle. *Lagenbeck's Arch Klin Chir* 1887;34:626–634.
33. Proetz AW. *Essays on the applied physiology of the nose.* St Louis: Annals Publishing, 1941;356.
34. Ritter FN. *The paranasal sinuses, anatomy and surgical technique.* St Louis: Mosby, 1973.
35. Bacher JA. Fatal air embolism after puncture of the maxillary antrum. *California Med* 1923;21:443.
36. Alden AM. A new procedure in the treatment of chronic maxillary sinus suppuration in children. *Arch Otolaryngol* 1926;4:521–525.
37. Asherson N. Intubation of the maxillary antrum for acute empyema. *Lancet* 1937;2:1399–1400.
38. Huggill PH, Ballantyne JC. An investigation into the relationship between adenoids and sinusitis in children. *J Otolaryngol* 1952;66:84–91.
39. Peterson RJ. Canine fossa puncture. *Laryngoscope* 1973;83:369–371.
40. Kim HN, Kim YM, Choi HS. Diagnostic and therapeutic significance of sinoscopy in maxillary sinusitis. *Yonsei Med J* 1985;26:59–67.
41. Stammberger H. *Functional endoscopic sinus surgery.* Philadelphia: BC Decker, 1991.
42. Spielberg W. Antroscopy of the maxillary sinus. *Laryngoscope* 1922;12:82.
43. St Clair T, Negus VE. *Diseases of the nose and throat.* 1937;232.
44. Maes JJ, Clement PA. The usefulness of irrigation of the maxillary sinus in children with maxillary sinusitis on the basis of the Waters' x-ray. *Rhinology* 1987;25:259–264.
45. Muntz HR, Lusk RP. Nasal antral windows in children: a retrospective study *Laryngoscope* 1990;100:643–646.
46. Hajek M. *Pathology and treatment of the inflammatory diseases of the nasal accessory sinuses.* St Louis: Mosby, 1926.
47. Hilding AC. Role of ciliary action in production of pulmonary atelectasis, vacuum in paranasal sinuses and in otitis media. *Ann Otol Rhinol Laryngol* 1943;52:816–833.
48. Freer OT. The antrum of Highmore: the removal of the greater part of its inner wall through the nostril for empyema. *Laryngoscope* 1905;15:343–349.
49. Sluder G. A modified Mikulicz operation whereby the entire lower turbinate is sawed in intranasal operations on the antrum of Highmore, with presentation of a patient. *Laryngoscope* 1909;19:904–910.
50. Canfield RB. The submucous resection of the lateral nasal wall in chronic empyema of the antrum, ethmoid and sphenoid. *JAMA* 1908;51:1136–1141.
51. Wilkerson WW. Antral window in the middle meatus. *Arch Ophthalmol* 1949;49:463–489.
52. Proetz AW. *The displacement method of sinus diagnosis and treatment.* St Louis: Annals Publishing, 1931;47.
53. Hilding AC. Experimental sinus surgery: effects of operative windows on normal sinuses. *Ann Otol Rhinol Laryngol* 1941;50:379–392.
54. Lavelle RJ, Harrison MS. Infection of the maxillary sinus: the case for the middle meatal antrostomy. *Laryngoscope* 1971;81:90–106.
55. Lang J. *Clinical anatomy of the nose, nasal cavity and paranasal sinuses.* New York: Thieme Medical Publishers, 1989;50–53.
56. Wigand ME. *Endoscopic surgery of the paranasal sinuses and anterior skull base.* New York: Thieme Medical Publishers, 1990.
57. Messerklinger W. *Endoscopy of the nose.* Baltimore: Urban & Schwarzenberg, 1978.
58. Stammberger H. Personal endoscopic operative technique for the lateral nasal wall—an endoscopic surgery concept in the treatment of inflammatory diseases of the paranasal sinuses. [Unsere endoskopische Operationstechnik der lateralen Nasenwand—ein endoskopisch-chirurgisches Konzept zur Behandlung entzundlicher Nasennebenhohlenerkrankungen.] *Laryngol Rhinol Otol (Stuttg)* 1985;64:559–566.
59. Messerklinger W. Uber die Drainage der menschlichen Nasennebenhohlen unter normalen und pathologischen Bedingungen. Second communication: Die Stirnhohlen und ihr Ausfuhrungssystem. *Monatsschr Ohrenheilkunde* 1967;101:313–326.
60. Wigand ME. Transnasal, endoscopical surgery for chronic sinusitis. III. Endonasal ethmoidectomy (author's translation). [Transnasale, endoskopische Chirurgie der Nasennebenhohlen bei chronischer Sinusitis. III. Die endonasale Siebbeinausraumung.] *HNO* 1981;29:287–293.
61. Wigand ME. Transnasal, endoscopical sinus surgery for chronic sinusitis. II. Endonasal operation of the maxillary antrum (author's translation). [Transnasale, endoskopische Chirurgie der Nasennebenhohlen bei chronischer Sinusitis. II. Die endonasale Kieferhohlen-Operation.] *HNO* 1981;29:263–269.
62. Panis R, Thumfart W, Wigand ME. Endonasal sinus surgery with endoscopic control for recurrent sinusitis in children (author's translation). [Die endonasale Kieferhohlenoperation mit endoskopischer Kontrolle als Therapie der chronisch rezidivierenden Sinusitis im Kindesalter.] *HNO* 1979;27:256–259.
63. Stammberger H. Endoscopic surgery for mycotic and chronic recurring sinusitis. *Ann Otol Rhinol Laryngol* 1985;119:1–11.
64. Kennedy DW. Serious misconceptions regarding functional endoscopic sinus surgery [letter]. *Laryngoscope* 1986;96:1170–1171.
65. Kennedy DW, Kennedy EM. Endoscopic sinus surgery. *AORN J* 1985;42:932–934.
66. Stankiewicz JA. Complications of endoscopic intranasal ethmoidectomy. *Laryngoscope* 1987;97:1270–1273.
67. Stankiewicz JA. Complications in endoscopic intranasal ethmoidectomy: an update. *Laryngoscope* 1989;99:686–690.
68. Buus DR, Tse DT, Farris BK. Ophthalmic complications of sinus surgery. *Ophthalmology* 1990;97:612–619.
69. Stankiewicz JA. Blindness and intranasal endoscopic ethmoidectomy: prevention and management. *Otolaryngol Head Neck Surg* 1989;101:320–329.
70. Freedman HM, Kern EB. Complications of intranasal ethmoidectomy: a review of 1,000 consecutive operations. *Laryngoscope* 1979;89:421–434.
71. Rosenbaum AL, Astle WF. Superior oblique and inferior rectus muscle injury following frontal and intranasal sinus surgery. *J Pediatr Ophthalmol* 1985;22:194–202.
72. Heinze JB, Hueston JT. Blindness after blepharoplasty: mechanism and early reversal. *Plast Reconstr Surg* 1978;61:347–354.
73. Hartley JH, Lester JC, Schatten WE. Acute retrobulbar hemorrhage during elective blepharoplasty. Its pathophysiology and management. *Plast Reconstr Surg* 1973;52:8–15.
74. Anderson RL, Edwards JJ. Bilateral visual loss after blepharoplasty. *Ann Plast Surg* 1980;5:288–292.
75. Walter RR. Is blindness a realistic complication in blepharoplasty procedures? *Ophthalmology* 1978;85:730–735.
76. Hayreh SS, Weingeist TA. Experimental occlusion of the central artery of the retina. IV: Retinal tolerance time to acute ischaemia. *Br J Ophthalmol* 1980;64:818–825.
77. Maniglia AJ, Chandler JR, Goodwin WJ, Flynn J. Rare complications following ethmoidectomies: a report of eleven cases. *Laryngoscope* 1981;91:1234–1244.
78. Anderson RL, Panje WR, Gross CE. Optic nerve blindness following blunt forehead trauma. *Ophthalmology* 1982;89:445–455.

Pediatric Sinusitis,
edited by R. P. Lusk,
Raven Press, Ltd., New York © 1992.

CHAPTER 11

Complications of Sinusitis

Rodney P. Lusk, Lawrence Tychsen, and T. S. Park

Acute and chronic sinusitis can cause significant morbidity and are potentially life threatening. The complications of sinusitis arise from extension of infection into the adjacent orbit or cranial vault.

ORBITAL CELLULITIS

In the preantibiotic era 1 in 5 patients (17 to 20%) with orbital cellulitis died from meningitis or had permanent loss of vision in the affected eye (1). The figure today is less than 5%. In acute cases of sinusitis with orbital cellulitis, temperatures greater than 38.5°C are frequently noted, the white blood cell (WBC) count is usually greater than 15,000 (2–4), recovery is usually longer, and there is a high rate of recurrence of the cellulitis. As a complication of sinusitis, orbital cellulitis occurs most frequently in the young (4,5). Fearon et al. (6) noted that 50% of the children in their series were under 6 years of age, and in the Hawkins and Clark series (7) 50% of the children were younger than 4. In general, younger children are successfully treated medically and older children are more likely to require surgical intervention (7).

Incidence

Orbital cellulitis is the most common complication of sinusitis and is most frequently associated with ethmoiditis (8–13). The incidence of infectious orbital complications secondary to sinusitis has been reported as 21% (11), 60% (9), 75% (14), and 90% (3). As Harrison (15) noted, sinusitis was not readily recognized in the preantibiotic era. Thus the orbital cellulitis literature from that era underreported associated sinusitis. Harrison estimates that the true figure correlating sinusitis with orbital cellulitis is approximately 70%. Some investigators have noted a higher frequency of infectious orbital complications during the winter and spring (12,16–18). The incidence appears to have stabilized over the past 2 decades (12,13).

Anatomy

The anatomic relationship between the sinuses and the orbit is the major factor in the pathogenesis of orbital cellulitis. The orbital wall is thinnest over the lamina papyracea (9,19) (lateral wall of the ethmoid sinus); paradoxically, the bone is less likely to be extremely thin in children than in adults (19). There are four possible routes by which ethmoid infection can extend into the orbit (Fig. 11.1):

1. *Venous.* Venous channels connect the orbital circulation with that of the ethmoid, frontal, and maxillary sinuses (14,20). The veins are sometimes referred to as the diploic veins of Breschet (21). They have no valves (9,22) and therefore provide an avenue of free communication between the two structures.
2. *Direct extension.* This occurs through bony dehiscences between the sinuses and orbit (14,19,23). The most likely site of dehiscence is in the lamina papyracea, as indicated by the predominance of subperiosteal abscesses in this location (24,25). For reasons that are not clear, subperiosteal abscess is more common on the left (3,11,12). In children, the frontal sinus is not well developed and its walls are not as thin. Therefore the chance of extension through the frontal bone to the orbit or brain is not as great, and the risk of meningitis is lower (26).

R. P. Lusk, L. Tychsen, and T. S. Park: Departments of Otolaryngology, Ophthalmology, and Neurosurgery, St. Louis Children's Hospital, St. Louis, Missouri 63110.

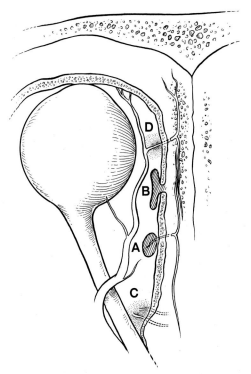

FIG. 11.1. Axial diagram of potential routes for expansion of infection from the ethmoid to the orbit. **A:** Venous. **B:** Direct extension. **C:** Lymphatic seeding. **D:** Arterial.

3. *Lymphatic seeding.* There are no lymph vessels within the orbit (9,22,27) and the lymphatic communication between sinus and orbit is limited. Thus lymphatic seeding is an unlikely mechanism.
4. *Arterial.* Spread is possible through this route; however, it is not thought to be an important factor.

Other Predisposing Factors

A number of extrinsic factors appear to predispose patients to sinusitis and the risk of orbital cellulitis. For example, swimmers have been noted in a prospective double-blind study, as well as retrospective studies, to have a higher incidence of sinusitis (8,28,29). A large number of studies report that nasal intubation in intensive care units increases the risk of sinusitis (30–39). Comatose head trauma patients also have a high rate of sinusitis, approximately 25%, with the maxillary sinus most frequently affected (40). Moloney et al. (8) documented that many types of facial infection can lead to orbital cellulitis. In fact, orbital complications may be associated with any infection of the face.

Signs and Symptoms

The signs and symptoms of orbital cellulitis associated with sinusitis can be used to help guide the management of the disease. The classification of orbital cellulitis in the literature is somewhat confusing. Some clinical investigators do not classify cases according to the location or extent of infection in the orbit but lump all types of inflammation (cellulitis to abscess) into one category (3,41). This makes it difficult to determine prognosis and the most effective medical and surgical therapy. For example, inflammation of the orbital contents without abscess formation can be treated successfully with antibiotics, but if an abscess occurs, antibiotics are much less successful and surgical drainage is more likely to be required.

In 1937, Hubert (42) classified orbital cellulitis of sinusitis into five categories of increasing severity:

1. Inflammatory edema of the eyelids with or without edema of the orbital contents (now commonly termed preseptal cellulitis).
2. Subperiosteal abscess with (a) edema of the eyelids and (b) spread of purulent exudate into the lid.
3. Abscess of the orbital tissues.
4. Mild and severe orbital cellulitis with phlebitis of the ophthalmic veins.
5. Cavernous sinus thrombosis.

In 1948, Smith and Spencer (43) presented a similar classification, which they used with a series of adult patients. They emphasized, however, that the categories are artificial divisions of what is really a continuum and are subject to change according to the severity of the disease. Chandler et al. (9), in 1970, modified the Smith–Spencer classification with the following schema, which has gained wide acceptance (10,41) (Fig. 11.2):

Group 1. Preseptal cellulitis—edema of the eyelids without tenderness and with no associated visual loss or limitation of extraocular motility (Figs. 11.2A and 11.3A–D).
Group 2. Orbital cellulitis without abscess—diffuse edema of the adipose tissues in the orbit with no abscess formation (Figs. 11.2B and 11.4A,B).
Group 3. Orbital cellulitis with subperiosteal abscess—abscess formation between the orbital periosteum and orbital bone; the abscess displaces the globe, usually down and laterally (14); if the proptosis is severe, it will be associated with limitation of ocular motility and perhaps decreased visual acuity (Figs. 11.2C and 11.5A,B).
Group 4. Orbital cellulitis with abscess within the orbital fat—proptosis is usually severe; proptosis may be purely frontally directed and not laterally or in-

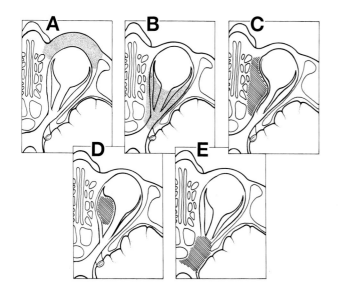

FIG. 11.2. Axial diagram of the progressive stages of inflammation of the orbit. **A:** Preseptal inflammation. **B:** Orbital cellulitis, involves the fat within the orbit. **C:** Subperiosteal abscess formation. **D:** Orbital abscess formation within fat and muscle cone. **E:** Cavernous sinus thrombosis.

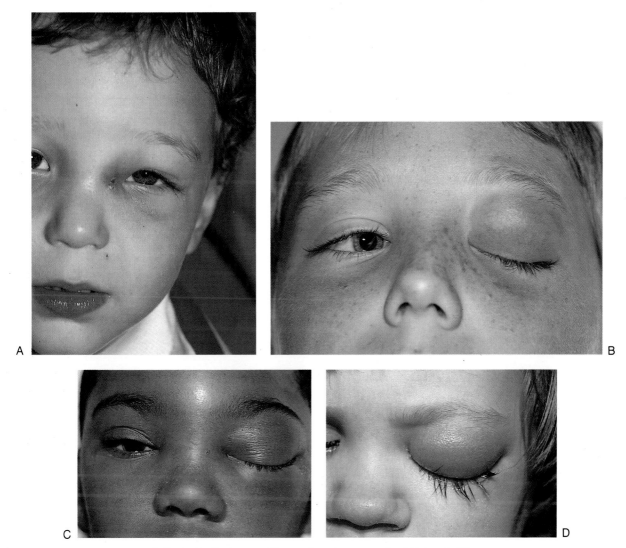

FIG. 11.3. Patients with varying degrees of orbital cellulitis.

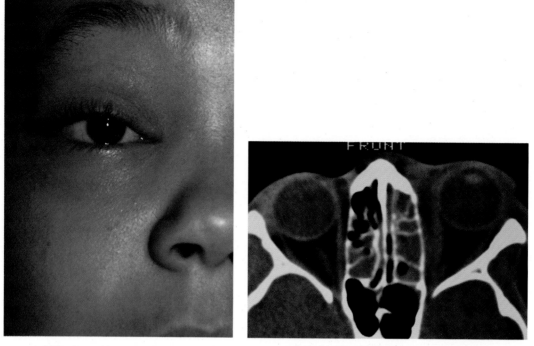

FIG. 11.4. A: Patient with cellulitis of the periosteum. **B:** Axial CT scan of patient

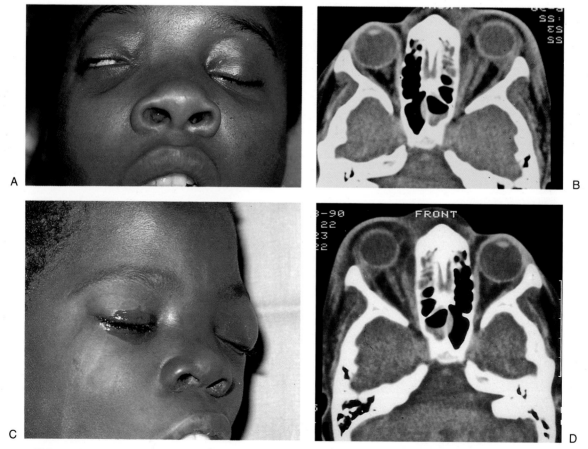

FIG. 11.5. A: Asymmetric proptosis secondary to subperiosteal abscess. **B:** CT scan of subperiosteal abscess. **C:** Another patient with asymmetric proptosis. **D:** CT scan of subperiosteal abscess.

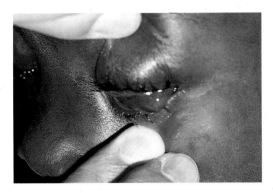

FIG. 11.6. Patient with chemosis of the eye secondary to an orbital infection.

feriorly displaced as in subperiosteal abscess; severe limitation of extraocular motility results (ophthalmoplegia) and visual loss due to optic neuropathy may ensue (in up to 13% of cases) (3) (Fig. 11.2D).
Group 5. Cavernous sinus thrombosis—orbital phlebitis extends into the cavernous sinus and across the basilar venous plexus to the opposite side, resulting in bilateral disease (Fig. 11.2E).

In each of these classification schemes, proptosis is a key diagnostic feature differentiating orbital cellulitis from preseptal cellulitis. Proptosis is present with any inflammatory reaction within the orbit and may be used as a crude indicator of abscess location. If the proptosis is symmetrical, the entire orbit is likely to be involved, but if it is asymmetrical the abscess is more likely to be located in the opposite orbital quadrant (Fig. 11.5A). In general, the greater the proptosis, the more severe the inflammation or the larger the abscess (9). Conjunctival swelling (chemosis) and ophthalmoplegia (causing diplopia) can occur with any expanding orbital mass (Fig. 11.6).

Loss of visual acuity is a symptom that demands prompt, accurate assessment. The most common cause of a decline in visual acuity in patients with or-

bital cellulitis is corneal refractive change, due to tear film disturbances, or astigmatism secondary to eyelid pressure. Limitation of motility, which is usually mechanical and caused by intraorbital edema, can also degrade vision by impeding accurate fixation on letter targets. When testing acuity, use of a pinhole, artificial teardrops, and free head movement are essential to separate these common causes of transient visual loss from true compressive optic neuropathy.

Compressive optic neuropathy (pressure on the nerve, its dural sheath, and its vascular supply) will always be accompanied by a relative afferent pupillary defect (Marcus Gunn pupil) (Fig. 11.7). Presence of a relative afferent pupillary defect is determined by the swinging flashlight test. The compressed nerve fails to transmit light impulses as readily as a normal nerve, resulting in a small amount of pupillary dilation when a flashlight is moved from the normal eye to the abnormal eye. The correlative symptom is the report by the patient that "someone turned down the lights" when looking monocularly through the eye with the compressed nerve.

Compression of the nerve compromises blood flow through the small perforating branches of the central retinal and ophthalmic arteries. The compression leads to decreased ophthalmic artery flow and hypoxic stasis of axoplasmic flow. If the nerve is compressed within 1.0 cm of the back of the globe, optic disc edema and engorgement of retinal veins can be seen (Fig. 11.8). Otherwise, no funduscopic sign may be evident. In rare cases in which orbital pressure reaches excessively high levels, central retinal artery flow may diminish or even cease. This is usually preceded by conspicuous pulsations of the large retinal arterioles on the optic disc. In this situation, emergent lateral canthotomy is indicated in preparation for orbital decompression. In human cases, and in monkey experiments, profound permanent visual loss is the rule if circulation is not restored within 100 min (44,45).

In patients who develop orbital cellulitis, 10% will

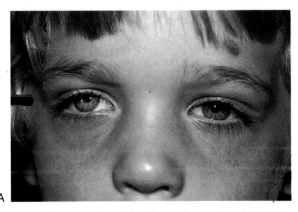
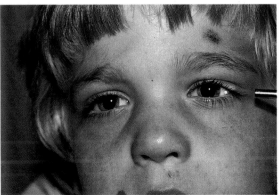

FIG. 11.7. Relative afferent pupillary defect in patient's left eye. **A:** Light shown in the right eye produces bilateral pupillary constriction. **B:** Light in left eye produces bilateral pupillary dilatation.

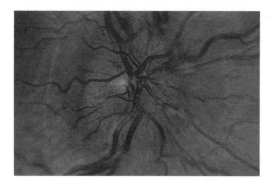

FIG. 11.8. Optic disc edema and engorgement of retinal veins.

It has been suggested that in ethmoiditis, the infection or inflammation process exerts direct pressure on the optic nerve. This mechanism would not account for optic neuropathy associated with maxillary sinusitis, and here it is hypothesized that infection or inflammation is more likely to spread through venous channels to the nerve sheath at the orbital apex (46). That the sinusitis is a major factor in the optic neuropathy is demonstrated by the finding that sinus drainage can produce rapid improvement in the vision in some cases (49). This suggests that immunoinflammatory products cause sludging and/or vasomotor changes that affect the optic nerve (46).

show at least a temporary decrease in visual acuity in the affected eye (11). The decrease may be bilateral and permanent if cavernous sinus thrombosis develops (44).

Optic nerve damage can occur not only from compressive ischemia but also from inflammation (inflammatory optic neuropathy). This is similar to, but distinct from, the demyelinating optic neuropathy (optic neuritis) of multiple sclerosis (46). Acute ethmoid sinus infection, mucoceles, pyoceles, and osteomyelitis have all been associated with inflammatory optic neuropathy (46–48).

Diagnostic Tests

If orbital cellulitis progresses rapidly or fails to respond to treatment with IV antibiotics, a subperiosteal abscess should be suspected. Clinically, it may be very difficult to distinguish between orbital cellulitis and subperiosteal abscess (8,12,13). Asymmetric proptosis (with the eye displaced away from the abscess) and asymmetric limitation of ocular motility are most frequently associated with subperiosteal abscess (Fig. 11.5B; see chapter by McAlister et al., Figs. 3.40–3.43). Diffuse orbital cellulitis is associated with sym-

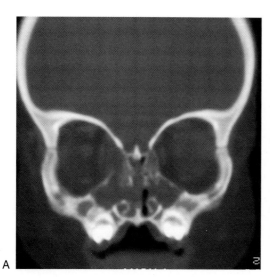

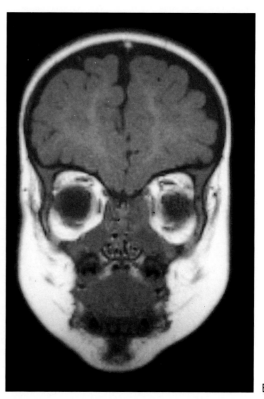

FIG. 11.9. A: Coronal CT scan of child with subperiosteal abscess of the right ethmoid sinus. **B:** MRI of same child.

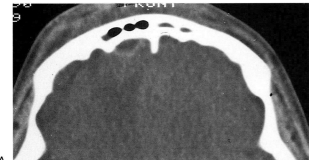
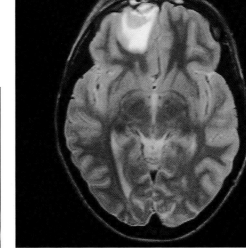

FIG. 11.10. A: CT scan of frontal lobe cerebritis associated with frontal and ethmoid sinusitis. **B:** MRI of same child with frontal lobe cerebritis; the cerebritis is more evident.

metrical (axial) proptosis and symmetrical limitation of ocular motility. Using these clinical criteria, the correct staging will be established in approximately 70% of the cases. CT scanning with contrast improves the correct staging to 82% (49). Moreover, CT scanning is the single best ancillary test to use in differentiating subperiosteal from orbital fat abscesses (8,12,16,49,50) (Fig. 11.5B; see chapter by McAlister et al., Fig. 3.42). It should be noted, however, that the correct staging will be ascertained only after surgery in approximately 20% of patients.

CT scans are recommended if the patient has not responded within 24 h to intravenous antibiotics (51); scans are imperative if periorbital abscess, orbital abscess, or cavernous sinus thrombosis is suspected clinically (4,49,51). CT scans are better than plain skull films in diagnosing chronic sinusitis (52) and in diagnosing orbital cellulitis in children (3,49). MRI is not particularly helpful in differentiating between orbital cellulitis and subperiosteal abscess (Fig. 11.9) but is helpful in those rare cases in which frontal lobe cerebritis is suspected (Fig. 11.10; see chapter by McAlister et al., Fig. 3.46).

Few patients with orbital cellulitis present with seizures or signs of meningismus (53,54); therefore its use as a routine diagnostic tool is not warranted (26). However, lumbar puncture is recommended in children who develop a fever and seizure episodes but only after CT or MRI scans have been obtained to rule out an abscess (55).

Microbiology

The organisms causing orbital cellulitis are associated with different sites of origin. Cellulitis of the face and septal cellulitis are most frequently caused by *Streptococcus* or *Staphylococcus aureus* (2,11). These organisms are also more likely to be associated with preseptal cellulitis. Infections that originate in the sinuses are most likely caused by the bacteria implicated in acute sinusitis: *Streptococcus pneumoniae, Hemophilus influenzae, Moraxella catarrhalis*, and *Streptococcus pyogenes* (Table 11.1) (11,14,41,56–59). *Staphylococcus aureus* is implicated in all age groups but is less likely to be the causative agent in young children (4). Anaerobes are unusual in acute infections (59).

Bacteremia in conjunction with orbital cellulitis is more common in young children (3,11,41). One study

TABLE 11.1. *Incidence of organisms causing acute sinusitis*

Organism	Revonta (250)[a]	Wald (248)	Ylikoski (1231)
Streptococcus pneumoniae	31%	36%	18.5%
Hemophilus influenzae	24%	23%	50.7%
Moraxella catarrhalis	2%	19%	1%
Streptococcus pyogenes	2%	2%	5%
Anaerobes			1.5%

[a] Number of cases in parentheses.

TABLE 11.2. *Antibiotic therapy for sinusitis and/or orbital cellulitis*

Clinical diagnosis	Initial choice	Alternatives
Sinusitis, acute	Amox/ampicillin or erythromycin + sulfonamide	Amox/clav,[a] cefaclor, cefuroxime, TMP-SMX[b]
Sinusitis, chronic	Antistaphylococcal or augmented penicillin	Cephalosporin, clindamycin
Orbital cellulitis	Ceftriaxone or cefotaxime or ceftazidime	Antistaphylococcal penicillin or vancomycin plus aztreonam or amox plus chloramphenicol

[a] Amox/clav, augmented amoxicillin/K⁺ clavulanate.

[b] TMP-SMX, trimethoprim–sulfamethoxazole.

reports a 30% incidence in patients less than 5 years old, 16% in those 4 to 8 years old, but less than 5% among adolescents and adults (4). This may be due to the inability of the young child to mount an appropriate antibody response to bacteria coated with polysaccharide capsules. For a more extensive discussion of this subject see the chapter by Muntz and Lusk.

Medical Management

Management of orbital cellulitis requires the expertise of many specialists: an otolaryngologist, an ophthalmologist, and a pediatrician versed in management of infectious disease. At the St. Louis Children's Hospital, these cases are best co-managed by an otolaryngologist–ophthalmologist duo since the sinusitis is best managed by the otolaryngologist, but the devastating complications are all visual (56). Medical management begins with administration of high-dose intravenous antibiotics capable of crossing the blood–brain barrier (14). Potential antibiotics are listed in Table 11.2. Steroids should be avoided because of the potential for complications (21). Nasal vasoconstrictors—Neo-synephrine, oxymetazoline, or even cocaine—should be used acutely (8). The patient's mental status, ocular motility, and visual acuity must be monitored closely. If the patient fails to improve or if there is progression of any of the symptoms, a CT scan should be obtained and in most cases the sinuses and orbit should be explored without delay.

Surgical Management

Previous reports show a wide variation in the number of patients with orbital cellulitis who will require surgical drainage—12 to 98%, with an average of 60% (4,7,16,60). Much of this variation is attributed to differences in patient ages and referral patterns. However, in the older child, it is more likely that medical management will fail and surgical management will be required (16).

At the St. Louis Children's Hospital, we follow an algorithm to help decide when or if to proceed to surgical drainage (Fig. 11.11). Cases vary and therapy must be individualized. Once a presumptive diagnosis of preseptal or orbital cellulitis is made, the child is admitted for IV antibiotic therapy and monitoring of visual and systemic signs. In general, if the disease has progressed, or if there is no improvement after 24 h of intravenous antibiotic therapy, or if there is an abrupt decline in the patient's clinical status, then a CT scan and/or MRI is obtained. If there is a nonrefractive decrease in visual acuity, accompanied by a relative afferent pupillary defect, then immediate surgical intervention should be implemented. As shown in the algorithm, we prefer coronal CT before abscess drainage. The coronal CT provides better three-dimensional localization of abscess size and relationship to globe, extraocular muscles, and optic nerve.

If an orbital abscess is evident on CT scan, then an orbitotomy (decompression of the abscess) with drainage of the ethmoid sinus is undertaken. It is very unusual to have a periorbital abscess without associated ethmoid disease. The ethmoid disease should be surgically removed at the time the subperiorbital abscess is drained. However, if there is extensive bleeding, the ethmoidectomy may be staged. The conventional method of ethmoidectomy and drainage of the abscess is through an external (Lynch) incision (Fig. 11.12A–D).

An experienced endoscopic sinus surgeon may attempt endoscopic drainage of a subperiosteal abscess by penetrating the lamina papyracea. This involves the standard endoscopic approach as described in the chapter by Lusk. The lamina papyracea is exposed throughout the length of the anterior and posterior ethmoids (see Figs. 10.53, 10.54, and 10.59 in Lusk chapter). Because of acute inflammation secondary to the infection, there will be more extensive bleeding and poorer visualization. Patience is required during repeated applications of topical vasoconstrictors. For these reasons, the endoscopic approach should be undertaken only by the most experienced endoscopic sur-

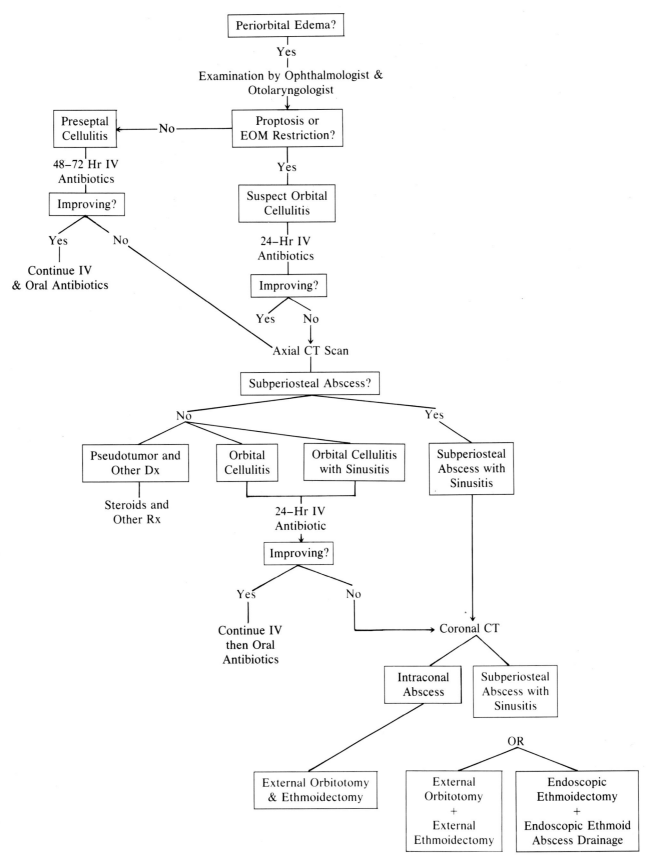

FIG. 11.11. St. Louis Children's algorithm for orbital cellulitis.

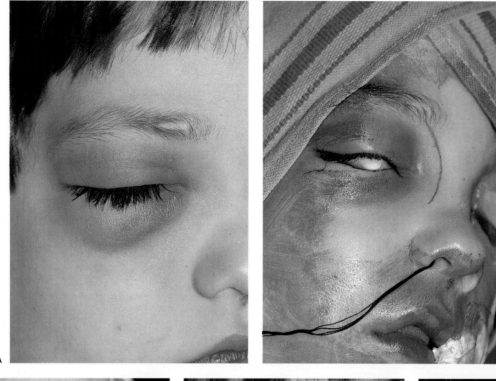

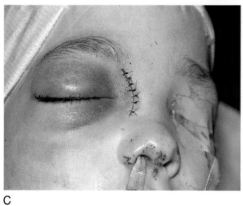

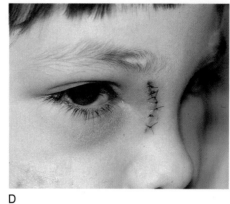

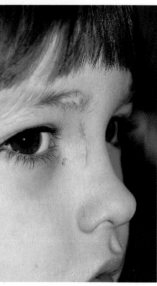

FIG. 11.12. A: Patient with preseptal inflammation and edema secondary to a sub-periosteal abscess. **B:** Patient in the operating room with the Lynch incision marked out. **C:** Incision closed. **D:** Incision and eye at 1 week postoperatively. **E:** Incision at approximately 4 weeks.

geons with the intention of readily converting to the external procedure if visualization is not adequate (Fig. 11.12). Only after the lamina papyracea is completely exposed should it be penetrated. If it is penetrated earlier, fat can herniate into the ethmoid cavity and obstruct the remainder of the dissection. The lamina papyracea is palpated and carefully penetrated at its thinnest point with a J curette or spoon (Fig. 11.13). The lamina papyracea will usually be thinnest anteriorly and therefore penetrated here first. When purulence is obtained it is cultured and the lamina papyracea is widely removed and the abscess drained.

Cavernous Sinus Inflammation With or Without Thrombosis

Orbital cellulitis or sphenoethmoiditis can extend posteriorly, causing inflammation of the venous cavernous sinus (Fig. 11.2E) (61,62). The earliest clinical symptoms of cavernous sinus thrombosis are headache and painful paresthesia in the distribution of the trigeminal nerve. Nasal discharge is usually present (63–65). Acute sphenoid sinusitis is frequently overlooked and the delayed diagnosis increases the chance of developing cavernous sinus thrombosis (see Fig. 10.64A

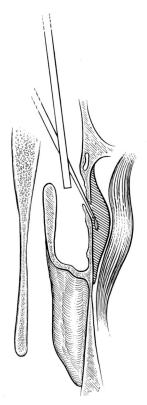

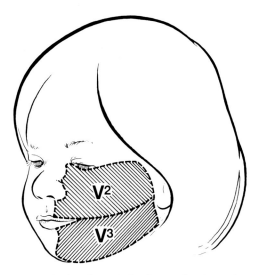

FIG. 11.15. Distribution of the hypesthesia and paraesthesia associated with trigeminal involvement.

FIG. 11.13. Axial diagram of a J curette piercing the lamina papyracea anteriorly to drain a subperiosteal abscess. The anatomical orientation is explained in Fig. 10.15A of the chapter by Lusk.

of chapter by Lusk) (65). Delayed diagnosis of cavernous involvement often leads to devastating neurological complications. The majority (66%) of patients are younger than 20 years (66).

Inflammatory pressure within the cavernous sinus can affect any of the cranial nerves (II to VI) coursing through it (Fig. 11.14). Venous pressure in the sinus is rarely high enough to compromise optic nerve perfusion, but inflammation of the nerve disrupts axoplasmic flow and can cause a relative afferent pupillary defect. More commonly, extraocular motility palsy is

caused by pressure and inflammation around the abducens nerve (which hugs the carotid) or on the lateral wall of the sinus, which contains the oculomotor and trochlear nerves (61,67) (Fig. 11.14).

The cranial nerve palsy may be masked by mechanical limitation of eye movement secondary to orbital edema or abscess. Visual acuity deficits or deficits in ocular motility may be permanent in up to 50% of cases of cavernous sinus thrombosis and up to 20% of cases of sphenoid sinusitis (63,65). The ophthalmic and maxillary division of the trigeminal nerve may be inflamed, resulting in hypesthesia and paraesthesia of the cornea, skin, and mucosa (Fig. 11.15).

An important diagnostic sign is sudden development of *bilateral* orbital disease (66,68). This is attributed to propagation of infection to the opposite side through the cavernous sinus plexus on the clivus and sella. Infection can then spread to dural sinuses and extend to the cortical and parenchymal veins (65,69,70), leading to meningitis and multiple cerebral venous thrombosis.

Lumbar puncture and culture of spinal fluid are war-

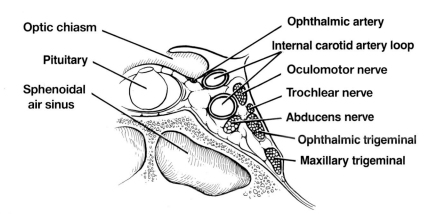

Optic chiasm
Pituitary
Sphenoidal air sinus
Ophthalmic artery
Internal carotid artery loop
Oculomotor nerve
Trochlear nerve
Abducens nerve
Ophthalmic trigeminal
Maxillary trigeminal

FIG. 11.14. Diagram of cranial nerves in the cavernous sinus.

ranted in the septic patient. If cavernous sinus thrombosis or related intracranial complications are suspected, emergent CT or MRI scanning is indicated. The lumbar puncture is performed after the scan to exclude patients at risk for tonsillar herniation with unrecognized brain abscess.

Cavernous sinus thrombosis on CT scan is evident as a lack of contrast enhancement in one or both cavernous sinuses. Coronal and axial CT of the sphenoid and ethmoid sinuses should be obtained at the same time (71). The axial CT scan is important to define the anatomical relationship between the sphenoid and the optic nerve and cavernous sinus.

The most common causative organisms in sphenoid sinusitis are *Staphylococcus aureus*, *Streptococcus pneumoniae*, and other aerobic or anaerobic streptococci (63,65,66).

Intravenous antibiotic therapy with a third-generation cephalosporin such as cefotaxime (72) is chosen to combat gram-positive cocci (*Staphylococcus*) and gram-negative bacilli. If the sinuses are opacified on CT they should be drained. Drainage of the sphenoid and ethmoid sinuses should be accomplished using the safest method for the individual surgeon and his or her skills.

In general, the older the patient the more likely the need for sphenoethmoidectomy (66). Also, the longer it takes to establish the diagnosis, the greater the chance that surgery will be needed. In the preantibiotic era mortality rates of 50% were recorded if the patient progressed to cavernous sinus thrombosis. Current mortality rates are 10 to 27% (6,65).

INTRACRANIAL COMPLICATIONS

Intracranial complications include meningitis and epidural and subdural brain abscess, which can be either acute or chronic. Intracranial complications from paranasal sinusitis, which appear most commonly in adolescent males (73,74), are exceeded in incidence only by orbital complications (75,76). The current overall incidence is probably between 3.7% (77) and 17% (73), although Sable et al. (78) report an incidence between 20 and 40%.

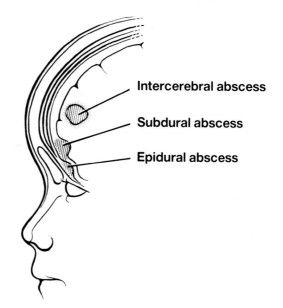

FIG. 11.16. Diagram of the position of a subdural, epidural, and brain abscess.

Brain abscesses, the most common complication (79), usually result from head and neck infections (21,68). In the past the most frequent source of brain abscess was the ear (80) but more recently it appears to be the sinuses (21,72,81–83). Brain abscesses have also been associated with congenital heart disease (84). The most common form of abscess is subdural, followed closely by frontal lobe abscess or a combination of the two (85) (Fig. 11.16). The overall incidence of paranasal sinusitis as a cause of frontal lobe abscess, however, is thought to be decreasing (86). Intracranial sequelae are most likely to occur in adults (73,87–89) and the incidence varies with location of the abscess (Table 11.3). Brain abscess appears to be rare in infants, with only 60 cases reported in the world literature (89); it is much more frequent in children older than 10 years (73).

Meningitis occurs most frequently in acute sphenoid sinusitis. A high index of suspicion is necessary to detect early meningitis and sinusitis as its source. Clues come from a thorough physical and neurological evaluation. If an abscess is suspected, a CT or MRI scan

TABLE 11.3. *Incidence of intracranial infections with sinusitis*

Study (number of cases)	Incidence of intracranial infections associated with sinusitis	Country
Yang, 1979 (1367)	0.5%	China
McClelland, 1978 (1368)	7.5%	Northern Ireland
Morgan, 1973 (1369)	9%	United States
Bradley and Shaw, 1983 (143)	15.7%	England
Van Alphen and Dreissen, 1976 (1371)	24%	The Netherlands
Snell, 1978 (1372)	24%	Canada

should be obtained before a lumbar puncture is performed to decrease the chance of tonsillar herniation (Fig. 11.10). Lew et al. (65) noted that 14 of 15 adult patients with acute sinusitis developed intracranial complications, but this seems unusually high. Meningitis can develop from sinusitis through direct extension or through interconnecting veins, primarily around the sphenoid sinus. Inflammation within the sphenoid sinus causes parameningeal inflammation of the cavernous sinus or direct infection of the veins, resulting in a cavernous sinus thrombosis. Veins of this region drain into dural sinuses, which can feed directly into the CSF to cause meningitis.

Signs and Symptoms

Brain abscesses are most likely to occur in the frontal lobes (Fig. 11.10). In this location they are particularly silent (90) and may be difficult to diagnosis on clinical grounds (80,85). Many patients—especially infants with open sutures that allow the brain to expand—do not necessarily develop signs of increased intracranial pressure (84).

Initially, brain abscesses cause symptoms similar to those of meningitis, but patients become less toxic in the subacute and chronic stages (91).

Symptoms of intracranial pressure include bradycardia, papilledema (which may not be present since it takes some time to develop) (85,92), stiff neck (73,85), hypertension, nausea, vomiting, and decreased consciousness (68). A dilated pupil is an ominous sign suggesting transtentorial herniation (93). Common symptoms of intracranial abscess include fever, headache, behavioral changes, seizures, nuchal rigidity, focal neurologic signs, and occasionally photophobia (73,79). A patient with epidural abscess generally presents with a continuous dull headache, sudden elevation of temperature, and normal CSF (88,91). A patient with a subdural abscess is usually toxic, with changes in mental status, severe headaches, nuchal rigidity, focal neurologic changes, papilledema, and cloudy CSF with leukocytes but no bacteria or positive cultures (88,91).

Fever and leukocytosis are frequently present with brain abscesses (73,85). There is a predominance of polymorphonuclear leukocytes and immature forms of white cells (73). Lumbar punctures, in cases of suspected brain abscess, are neither diagnostic nor helpful, and the risk of brain stem herniation far outweighs potential benefits (73,88). The lumbar puncture should only be performed after a CT scan or MRI has been performed to rule out a mass that could result in herniation. When a lumbar puncture is performed, the protein level (94) and white blood count may be elevated (87). Subdural abscesses are felt to be the most

dangerous intracranial complications and require emergent surgery (88). Three of seven patients with subdural abscesses died in the series of Maniglia et al. (21).

Diagnostic Imaging

CT scanning with contrast has been the test of choice (73,75,95–98) in the diagnosis and monitoring of medical therapy for brain abscesses; however, magnetic resonance imaging (MRI) holds promise for detecting early cellulitis and small abscesses (Fig. 11.10).

Several authors (99–102) have reported the failure of CT scans to reliably identify acute extra-axial empyemas. Weingarten et al. (99) observed that MRI was superior to CT in detecting small epidural and subdural abscesses in 5 of 6 adult patients and equivalent in the sixth. They also claimed that the MRI could unequivocally differentiate between epidural and subdural abscesses, which the CT scan could not, and differentiate purulence from other lesions such as sterile effusions and hematomas (99). Thus MRI appears to be more sensitive and localizes and delineates the disease more accurately.

MRI can also be used to rule out an abscess or mass prior to performing a lumbar puncture. This differentiation is important because early detection allows earlier medical and surgical intervention. The high morbidity and mortality rates associated with these violent yet curable infections are in large part due to the inability of CT scans to distinguish the lesion.

Microbiology

Intracranial complications are most frequently secondary to ear and sinus infections; therefore the most common organisms to be involved are those that occur in these areas. Acute suppurative otitis media is usually caused by *S. pneumoniae*, *Hemophilus influenza*, and *Moraxella catarrhalis* and is found most commonly in the young (4,6,7,41,103). Over the past 50 years there has been a steady increase in the proportion of *Hemophilus* infections and a progressive decline in streptococcal otitis media (*Streptococcus pyogenes* and beta-hemolytic group A *Streptococcus*). Acute mastoiditis is most often caused by *S. pneumoniae*, closely followed by *Streptococcus pyogenes* and *S. aureus*. Chronic otitis media and mastoiditis are associated with the same organisms but with a relatively higher incidence of *Staphylococcus aureus*. In acute sinusitis, the same pathogens are implicated as in ear infections, while in chronic sinusitis there is a much higher proportion of *S. aureus* and alpha-hemolytic streptococci (104,105).

In subdural abscesses (88), which are associated with sinusitis in 53% and otitis media in 12% of cases (83), *S. aureus* is the most common organism. Anaerobic bacteria have also been cultured and are thought by some investigators to be the primary causative agent of brain abscesses (21,106,107). Other bacteria that have been cultured are *Escherichia coli*, *Pseudomonas*, and *Proteus* (88,108,109). When the intracranial complication has occurred secondary to trauma, alpha-hemolytic streptococci, nonhemolytic streptococci, and *Staphylococcus aureus* are common (73,110).

Medical Management

Medical therapy must include antibiotics that cross the blood–brain barrier and cover the most frequently cultured bacteria. Different regimens have been proposed, including (a) cefuroxime (50 to 100 mg/kg/d) and metronidazole (30 mg/kg/d iv) (88), (b) chloramphenicol (75 to 100 mg/kg/d) and oxacillin (150 to 200 mg/kg/d) (73), or (c) until a specific etiology is identified, according to the John Nelson pocketbook of pediatric antimicrobial therapy, methicillin (200 mg/kg/d iv every 6 h), *and* aminoglycoside or cefotaxime (200 mg/kg/d iv every 6 h), *and* metronidazole (30 mg/kg/d iv every 8 h) (111). The duration of therapy is individualized. Johnson et al. (73) treated their patients for an average of 5 weeks, and Parker et al. (88) treated patients for 6 weeks. The patients' symptoms are followed, and serial CT scans are used to follow the lesion. If progression is seen, the abscess is drained, cultured, and treated according to antibiotic sensitivities.

Medical management alone has met with variable success. Johnson et al. (95) were not able to cure a single adult patient with medical therapy consisting mainly of chloramphenicol (75 to 100 mg/kg/d) and oxacillin (150 to 200 mg/kg/d). In following their patients sequentially with CT scans, they found that all the abscesses had progressed and all required surgical drainage. Exclusive medical management appears to be most appropriate in patients in the "cellulitis" stage of abscess formation (73,112,113).

Rennels et al. (113) concluded that antibiotics had the greatest chance of success if the lesion was small and the symptoms were of short duration. Johnson et al. (73) had four patients in this category who progressed to frank abscess formation in spite of aggressive IV medical management. These authors did not think that antibiotic choice was a factor since the organisms grown were sensitive to the antibiotics used.

Steroid therapy for intracranial and orbital infections is somewhat controversial (21). The rationale for it is to potentially inhibit capsule formation and collagen deposition (114–117). Steroids have been shown to interfere with antibiotic penetration and with the host's immunologic resistance (116,118,119), however, and their use in the treatment of intracranial infections is generally not recommended (21).

Surgical Management

Surgical management is based on the extent of disease in the involved structures. It is best orchestrated through a team approach, with complete exenteration of the diseased structures as a goal (88,91). Hoyt and Fisher (83) found that infections associated with mastoiditis *did not* require surgical drainage, but all those associated with sinusitis *did* require drainage. They also found that sinus drainage performed simultaneously with neurosurgical drainage significantly reduced the need for reexploration.

The intracranial approach is dictated by the location of the lesion. If the sinuses are involved, a craniofacial approach may be necessary to provide optimal exposure when disease of the paranasal sinuses has extended directly into the anterior cranial fossa. With the frontal sinus, endoscopy has altered the therapeutic approach. In the past when chronic disease had not eroded the posterior table of the frontal sinus, the sinus was cleared of all infection, the mucosa drilled from the bone, and abdominal fat harvested and placed into the sinus to obliterate it (120,121). Now the frontal sinus is increasingly approached from below, through the frontal recess, in an effort to improve the drainage from the frontal sinus.

Sequelae

Disabilities reported include seizures in 35%, blindness in 7.5%, and hemiparesis in 2% (85). Reported death rates range from 21% (21), 24% (85), 35.2% (96), to 15 to 43% (122). The older the patient with a brain abscess secondary to a sinus infection, the more likely a fatal outcome (85,123). The earlier the medical and surgical intervention, the better the chance of reducing disability and fatality rates.

POTT'S PUFFY TUMOR

Sir Percival Pott in 1775 described a well-circumscribed tumor of the forehead in patients with frontal sinusitis (124) (Fig. 11.17). In 1879 Lannelongue reported that Pott's puffy tumor was secondary to osteomyelitis of the anterior wall of the frontal sinus (125). The sinus mucosa and marrow of the frontal bone have a common venous drainage system of valveless diploic veins. A frontal sinus infection can invade

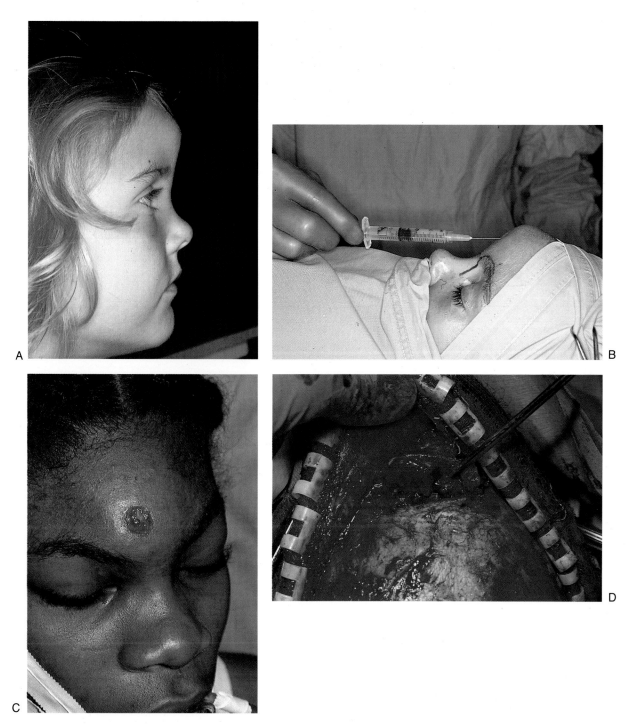

FIG. 11.17. A: Photo of patient with Pott's puffy tumor. **B:** Aspiration of purulence from the abscess. **C:** Another patient with a Pott's puffy tumor that includes breakdown of the skin. **D:** Coronal scalp flap is used to gain access to the sinus and purulent debris can be seen within the sinus.

the marrow cavity through these veins and cause osteomyelitis that erodes through the anterior table of the frontal bone (126). The erosion can also occur posteriorly, resulting in subdural empyema (86,127) (Fig. 11.18A–F; see Fig. 3.44 of chapter by McAlister et al.).

If the diploic veins become infected, a septic thrombophlebitis results, which can extend into the sagittal sinus, spread through the diploic veins into the CNS, and cause subdural empyema and brain abscess formation (126).

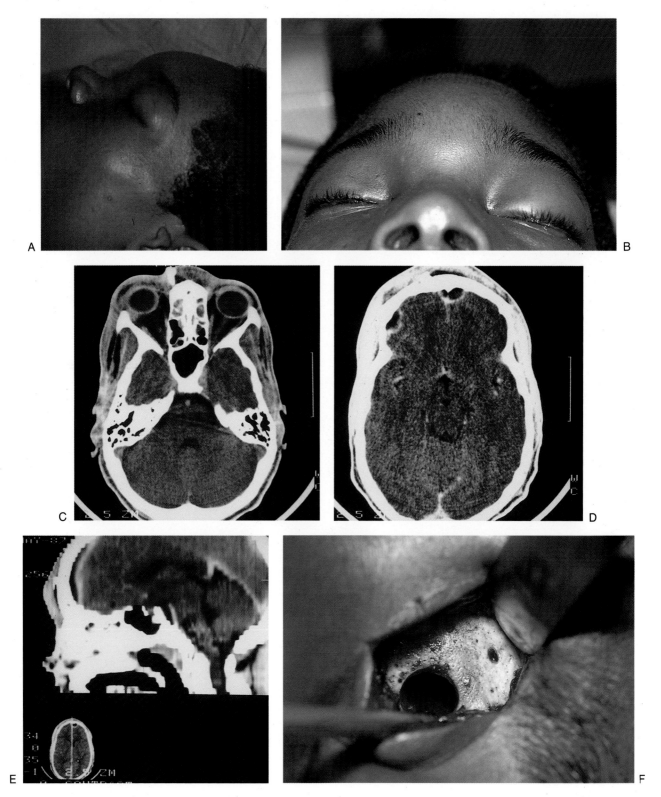

FIG. 11.18. A, B: Two views of a patient with a Pott's puffy tumor. **C, D:** Axial CT scans of patient. **E:** Reconstructed sagittal CT scan of patient A. **F:** A frontal sinus trephination is performed that shows purulence in the frontal sinus.

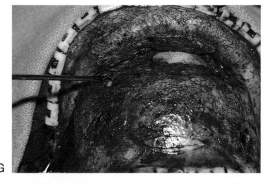

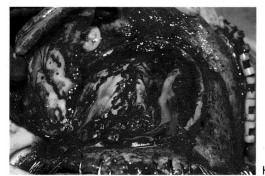

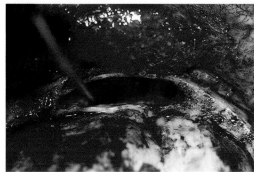

FIG. 11.18. (*Continued*) **G:** The coronal scalp flap is raised. **H:** There is extensive purulence secondary to a very large abscess over a large portion of the brain. **I:** The frontal sinus is cleaned of purulent debris but not obliterated. An ethmoidectomy is combined with the procedure.

The signs and symptoms of frontal sinusitis are often nonspecific, and differentiating them from infections in other sinuses may be difficult. Persistent pain and tenderness over the frontal area, which are suggestive of frontal sinusitis, are frequently absent (78). Subdural abscesses and frontal abscesses are frequently silent, and a high index of suspicion is necessary.

Radiologic studies are necessary to confirm the diagnosis of sinusitis. As noted in the chapter by McAlister et al., plain films, which show opacification, air–fluid levels, and mucosal thickening (128), do not adequately define the extent of disease. CT scans are more sensitive for detecting sinusitis (52,129,130) and its complications, such as osteomyelitis and CNS abscesses (131). CT scans with contrast are necessary to ensure that the infection has not extended posteriorly to form an intracranial cellulitis or abscess (126) (Fig. 11.10).

In Pott's puffy tumor, as in frontal sinusitis, *Staphylococcus aureus*, nonenterococcal streptococci, and oral anaerobes are the major causative organisms (126).

Intravenous therapy alone is not adequate to treat most cases of Pott's puffy tumor. Almost all will require aggressive surgical management (126). The contents of the frontal sinus should be cultured for anaerobic and aerobic bacteria, and antibiotic sensitivity tests should be performed. The antibiotics used should be the same as those for intracranial lesions (described in the intracranial section specifically covering streptococci and staphylococci). The antibiotics chosen, such as the third-generation cephalosporins, should have good CNS penetration (126). Specific therapy is altered based on the cultured organism. Antibiotics should be continued for 4 to 6 weeks to prevent osteomyelitis intracranial complications (131).

TOXIC SHOCK SYNDROME

Toxic shock syndrome, originally described by Todd et al. in 1978 (132), is a rare but potentially fatal complication of sinusitis. The children in the Todd et al. series had fever, multisystem failure, hypotension, and rash leading to desquamation. *S. aureus* was found in 5 of the 7 patients. In the spring and summer of 1980, widespread attention was focused on the disease because of an outbreak of cases in menstruating women using tampons. A significant number of cases are not associated with menses, however. It appears that any focus of staphylococcal infection can result in the syndrome (133,134). Toxic shock syndrome has been reported with influenza outbreaks but this is probably secondary to an associated *Staphylococcus aureus* infection of the sinuses (135).

A toxic shock-like syndrome has also been recognized in patients with streptococcal infections (136). The infections are usually associated with group A beta-hemolytic *Streptococcus* or *Streptococcus pyogenes*. These organisms are frequently found in pharyngitis, impetigo, erysipelas, necrotizing fasciitis, myositis, and bacteremia. The same syndrome is also thought to be associated with rheumatic fever, glomerulonephritis, and erythema nodosum. Ninety percent of the group A streptococcal organisms produce extracellular proteins called streptococcal pyrogenic exotoxins, which are designated A, B, and C (137–139). Johnson and L'Italien (140) found that exotoxin A and *S. aureus* enterotoxin B have in common a primary molecular structure with an amino acid homology of 50%. This probably accounts for the toxic-like symptoms in these streptococcal infections.

Toxic shock syndrome has been reported in children (141) and adults (136) secondary to sinusitis. In chronic sinusitis, *S. aureus* is frequently cultured from the nasal vestibule. The sinuses therefore can be a source of infection for toxic shock syndrome. Jacobson et al. (142) found nasal colonization of *S. aureus* in 35% of asymptomatic adults screened before elective surgery. Seven percent of these patients were toxic shock syndrome toxin-1-producing but none of the patients developed the syndrome. Osterholm and Kelly (143) found 11 of 22 healthy children harbored *S. aureus* in their nares with 4 of the 11 positive for toxic shock syndrome toxin-1-producing organisms. The initial step in the diagnostic workup should be a coronal CT scan followed by surgical drainage and culture of the sinus.

OTHER COMPLICATIONS

Additional complications of sinusitis such as asthma are discussed in other chapters.

REFERENCES

1. Gamble RC. Acute inflammation of the orbit in children. *Arch Ophthalmol* 1933;10:483–497.
2. Weizman Z, Mussaffi H. Ethmoiditis-associated periorbital cellulitis. *Int J Pediatr Otorhinolaryngol* 1986;11:147–151.
3. Weiss A, Friendly D, Eglin K, Chang M, Gold B. Bacterial periorbital and orbital cellulitis in childhood. *Ophthalmology* 1983;90:195–203.
4. Schramm VL Jr, Carter HD, Kennerdell JS. Evaluation of orbital cellulitis and results of treatment. *Laryngoscope* 1982;92:732–738.
5. Rubinstein JB, Handler SD. Orbital and periorbital cellulitis in children. *Head Neck Surg* 1982;5:15–21.
6. Fearon B, Edmonds B, Bird R. Orbital facial complications of sinusitis in children. *Laryngoscope* 1979;89:947–953.
7. Hawkins DB, Clark RW. Orbital involvement in acute sinusitis. Lessons from 24 childhood patients. *Clin Pediatr (Phila)* 1977;16:464–471.
8. Moloney JR, Badham NJ, McRae A. The acute orbit. Preseptal (periorbital) cellulitis, subperiosteal abscess and orbital cellulitis due to sinusitis. *J Laryngol Otol [Suppl]* 1987;12:1–18.
9. Chandler JR, Langenbrunner DJ, Stevens ER. The pathogenesis of orbital complications in acute sinusitis. *Laryngoscope* 1970;80:1414–1428.
10. Wald ER. Acute sinusitis and orbital complications in children. *Am J Otolaryngol* 1983;4:424–427.
11. Schramm VL Jr, Myers EN, Kennerdell JS. Orbital complications of acute sinusitis: evaluation, management, and outcome. *ORL J Otolaryngol Relat Spec* 1978;86:221–230.
12. Swift AC, Charlton G. Sinusitis and the acute orbit in children. *J Laryngol Otol* 1990;104:213–216.
13. Moloney JR, Badham NJ, McRae A. The acute orbit. Preseptal (periorbital) cellulitis, subperiosteal abscess and orbital cellulitis due to sinusitis. *J Laryngol Otol [Suppl]* 1987;12:1–18.
14. Goodwin WJ Jr. Orbital complications of ethmoiditis. *Otolaryngol Clin North Am* 1985;18:139–147.
15. Harrison HC. Orbital cellulitis with abscess formation caused by sinusitis [letter; comment]. *Ann Otol Rhinol Laryngol* 1989;98:322.
16. Welsh LW, Welsh JJ. Orbital complications of sinus diseases. *Laryngoscope* 1974;84:848–856.
17. Haynes RE, Cramblett HG. Acute ethmoiditis: its relationship to orbital cellulitis. *Am J Dis Child* 1967;114:261–267.
18. Guindi GM. Acute orbital cellulitis: a multidisciplinary emergency. *Br J Oral Maxillofac Surg* 1983;21:201–207.
19. Mills RP, Kartush JM. Orbital wall thickness and the spread of infection from the paranasal sinuses. *Clin Otolaryngol* 1985;10:209–216.
20. Batson OV. Relationship of the eye to the paranasal sinuses. *Arch Ophthalmol* 1936;16:322–323.
21. Maniglia AJ, Goodwin WJ, Arnold JE, Ganz E. Intracranial abscesses secondary to nasal, sinus, and orbital infections in adults and children. *Arch Otolaryngol Head Neck Surg* 1989;115:1424–1429.
22. Avery LB. The sense organs. In: Schaefer JP, ed. *Morris human anatomy*. New York: Blakiston, 1953;1152–1153.
23. Ritter FN. The maxillary sinus. In: Ritter FN, ed. *The paranasal sinuses: anatomy and surgical technique*. St Louis: Mosby, 1973.
24. Goldberg F, Berne AJ, Oski FA. Differential of orbital cellulitis from preseptal cellulitis by computed tomography. *Pediatrics* 1978;62:1000–1004.
25. Harris GJ. Subperiosteal abscess of the orbit. *Arch Ophthalmol* 1983;101:751–757.
26. Antoine GA, Grundfast KM. Periorbital cellulitis. *Int J Pediatr Otorhinolaryngol* 1987;13:273–278.
27. Basmasion JV. Orbital cavity and contents. In: Basmasion JV, ed. *Grant's method of anatomy*, 9th ed. Baltimore: Williams & Wilkins, 1975;500.
28. Deitmer T, Scheffler R. Nasal physiology in swimmers and swimmers' sinusitis. *Acta Otolaryngol (Stockh)* 1990;110:286–291.
29. Healy GB, Strong MS. Acute periorbital swelling. *Laryngoscope* 1972;82:1491–1498.
30. Pedersen J, Schurizek BA, Melsen NC, Juhl B. Sinusitis caused by nasotracheal intubation [in Danish]. *Ugeskr Laeger* 1990;152:379–381.
31. Fassoulaki A. Nasotracheal intubation, paranasal sinusitis and head injuries [letter]. *Br J Anaesth* 1989;62:236–237.
32. Lëvy C, Meyer P, Guërin JM, Deberardinis F, Aouala D. Nosocomial sinusitis in an intensive care unit. Role of nasotracheal intubation [in French]. *Ann Otolaryngol Chir Cervicofac* 1988;105:549–552.
33. Miner JD, Elliott CL, Johnson CW, McSoley T, Spahn JG, Spahn T. Nosocomial sinusitis. *Indiana Med* 1988;81:684–686.
34. Hansen M, Poulsen MR, Bendixen DK, Hartmann-Andersen F. Incidence of sinusitis in patients with nasotracheal intubation. *Br J Anaesth* 1988;61:231–232.
35. Linden BE, Aguilar EA, Allen SJ. Sinusitis in the nasotracheally intubated patient. *Arch Otolaryngol Head Neck Surg* 1988;114:860–861.
36. Meyer PH, Guerin JM. Acute paranasal sinusitis and nasotracheal intubation [letter]. *Crit Care Med* 1988;16:206.
37. Guerin JM, Meyer P, Habib Y. Nosocomial pneumonia and sinusitis in intubated intensive care unit patients [letter]. *Am Rev Respir Dis* 1987;136:1310.
38. Grindlinger GA, Niehoff J, Hughes SL, Humphrey MA, Simpson G. Acute paranasal sinusitis related to nasotracheal intubation of head-injured patients. *Crit Care Med* 1987;15:214–217.

39. Fougeront B, Bodin L, Lamas G, Bokowy C, Elbez M. Sinusitis during intensive care. Prospective studies [in French]. *Ann Otolaryngol Chir Cervicofac* 1990;107:329–332.

40. Humphrey MA, Simpson GT, Grindlinger GA. Clinical characteristics of nosocomial sinusitis. *Ann Otol Rhinol Laryngol* 1987;96:687–690.

41. Shapiro ED, Wald ER, Brozanski BA. Periorbital cellulitis and paranasal sinusitis: a reappraisal. *Pediatr Infect Dis* 1982;1:91–94.

42. Hubert L. Orbital infections due to nasal sinusitis. *NY State J Med* 1937;37:1559.

43. Smith AT, Spencer JT. Orbital complications resulting from lesions of the sinuses. *Ann Otol Rhinol Laryngol* 1948;57:5–27.

44. Anderson RL, Edwards JJ. Bilateral visual loss after blepharoplasty. *Ann Plast Surg* 1980;5:288–292.

45. Hayreh SS, Weingeist TA. Experimental occlusion of the central artery of the retina. IV: Retinal tolerance time to acute ischaemia. *Br J Ophthalmol* 1980;64:818–825.

46. Awerbuch G, Labadie EL, Van Dalen JT. Reversible optic neuritis secondary to paranasal sinusitis. *Eur Neurol* 1989;29:189–193.

47. Rothstein J, Maisel RH, Berlinger NT, Wirtschafter JD. Relationship of optic neuritis to disease of the paranasal sinuses. *Laryngoscope* 1984;94:1501–1508.

48. Simpson DE, Moser LA. Compressive optic neuropathy secondary to chronic sinusitis. *Am J Optom Physiol Opt* 1988;65:757–762.

49. Gutowski WM, Mulbury PE, Hengerer AS, Kido DK. The role of CT scans in managing the orbital complications of ethmoiditis. *Int J Pediatr Otorhinolaryngol* 1988;15:117–128.

50. Bilaniuk LT, Zimmerman RA. Computer-assisted tomography: sinus lesions with orbital involvement. *Head Neck Surg* 1980;2:293–301.

51. Wald ER, Pang D, Milmoe GJ, Schramm VL Jr. Sinusitis and its complications in the pediatric patient. *Pediatr Clin North Am* 1981;28:777–796.

52. McAlister WH, Lusk RP, Muntz HR. Comparison of plain radiographs and coronal CT scans in infants and children with recurrent sinusitis. *Am J Roentgenol* 1989;153:1259–1264.

53. Lober J, Sunderland R. Lumbar puncture in children with convulsions associated with fever. *Lancet* 1980;1:785–786.

54. Rutler N, Smales ORC. Role of routine investigations in children presenting with their first febrile convulsion. *Arch Dis Child* 1977;52:188–191.

55. Oullette EM. The child who convulses with fever. *Pediatr Clin North Am* 1974;21:467–481.

56. Robie G, O'Neal R, Kelsey DS. Periorbital cellulitis. *J Pediatr Ophthalmol* 1977;14:354–363.

57. Revonta M, Suonpaa J. Diagnosis of subacute maxillary sinusitis in children. *J Laryngol Otol* 1981;95:133–140.

58. Wald ER, Milmoe GJ, Bowen A, Ledesma-Medina J, Salamon N, Bluestone CD. Acute maxillary sinusitis in children. *N Engl J Med* 1981;304:749–754.

59. Ylikoski J, Savolainen S, Jousimies-Somer H. The bacteriology of acute maxillary sinusitis. *ORL J Otorhinolaryngol Relat Spec* 1989;51:175–181.

60. Noel LP, Clarke WN, Peacocke RA. Periorbital and orbital cellulitis in childhood. *Can J Ophthalmol* 1981;16:178–180.

61. Karlin RJ, Robinson AL Jr. Septic cavernous sinus thrombosis. *Ann Emerg Med* 1984;13:449–455.

62. Shaw RE. Cavernous sinus thrombophlebitis: a review. *Br J Surg* 1952;40:40–47.

63. Wyllie JW, Kern EB, Djalilian M. Isolated sphenoid sinus lesions. *Laryngoscope* 1973;83:1252–1265.

64. Abramovich S, Smelt GJ. Acute sphenoiditis, alone and in concert. *J Laryngol Otol* 1982;96:751–757.

65. Lew D, Southwick FS, Montgomery WW. Sphenoid sinusitis: a review of 30 cases. *N Engl J Med* 1983;309:1149–1154.

66. Shahin J, Gullane PJ, Dayal VS. Orbital complications of acute sinusitis. *J Otolaryngol* 1987;16:23–27.

67. Weisberger EC, Dedo HH. Cranial neuropathies in sinus disease. *Laryngoscope* 1977;87:357–363.

68. Harrington PC. Complications of sinusitis. *Ear Nose Throat J* 1984;63:163–171.

69. Caplan LR. Vertebrobasilar occlusive disease. In: Barnett HJM, Mohr JR, Stein BM, eds. *Pathophysiology, diagnosis, and management.* New York: Churchill Livingstone, 1986;549–619.

70. Smith BH. Infections of the cranial dura and the dural sinuses. In: Vinken PJ, Bruyn GW, eds. *Handbook of clinical neurology.* Amsterdam: North-Holland, 1991;149–186.

71. Rao KC, Knipp HC, Wagner EJ. Computed tomographic findings in cerebral sinus and venous thrombosis. *Radiology* 1981;140:391–398.

72. Macdonald RL, Findlay JM, Tator CH. Sphenoethmoidal sinusitis complicated by cavernous sinus thrombosis and pontocerebellar infarction. *Can J Neurol Sci* 1988;15:310–313.

73. Johnson DL, Markle BM, Wiedermann BL, Hanahan L. Treatment of intracranial abscesses associated with sinusitis in children and adolescents. *J Pediatr* 1988;113:15–23.

74. Kaufman DM, Litman N, Miller MH. Sinusitis: induced subdural empyema. *Neurology* 1983;33:123–132.

75. Dietrich U, Feldges A, Nau HE, Löhr E. Epidural abscess following frontal sinusitis—demonstration of communication by epidural contrast medium and coronal computerized tomography. *Comput Med Imaging Graph* 1989;13:351–354.

76. Kaufman DM, Miller MH, Steigbigel NH. Subdural empyema: analysis of 17 recent cases and review of the literature. *Medicine (Baltimore)* 1975;54:485–498.

77. Clayman GL, Adams GL, Paugh DR, Koopmann CF Jr. Intracranial complications of paranasal sinusitis: a combined institutional review. *Laryngoscope* 1991;101:234–239.

78. Sable NS, Hengerer A, Powell KR. Acute frontal sinusitis with intracranial complications. *Pediatr Infect Dis* 1984;3:58–61.

79. Harris LF, Haws FP, Triplett JN Jr, Maccubbin DA. Subdural empyema and epidural abscess: recent experience in a community hospital. *South Med J* 1987;80:1254–1258.

80. Pennybaker J. Abscess of the brain. In: *Modern trend in neurology.* London: Butterworth, 1951;251–290.

81. Bradley PJ, Shaw MD. Three decades of brain abscess on Merseyside. *J R Coll Surg* 1983;28:223–228.

82. Snell GE. Sinogenic and otogenic brain abscess. *J Otolaryngol* 1978;7:289–296.

83. Hoyt DJ, Fisher SR. Otolaryngologic management of patients with subdural empyema. *Laryngoscope* 1991;101:20–24.

84. Spires JR, Smith RJ, Catlin FI. Brain abscesses in the young. *Otolaryngol Head Neck Surg* 1985;93:468–474.

85. Bradley PJ, Manning KP, Shaw MD. Brain abscess secondary to paranasal sinusitis. *J Laryngol Otol* 1984;98:719–725.

86. Remmler D, Boles R. Intracranial complications of frontal sinusitis. *J Laryngol Otol* 1980;90:1814–1824.

87. Rosenbaum AL, Astle WF. Superior oblique and inferior rectus muscle injury following frontal and intranasal sinus surgery. *J Pediatr Ophthalmol* 1985;22:194–202.

88. Parker GS, Tami TA, Wilson JF, Fetter TW. Intracranial complications of sinusitis. *South Med J* 1989;82:563–569.

89. Zellers TM, Donowitz LG. Brain abscess and ethmoid sinusitis presenting as periorbital cellulitis in a two-month-old infant. *Pediatr Infect Dis J* 1987;6:213–215.

90. Liston ED, Walikerle JF, Robinson W. Intracranial abscess with behavioral changes. *Arch Otolaryngol* 1979;105:343–346.

91. Morgan PR, Morrison WV. Complications of frontal and ethmoid sinusitis. *Laryngoscope* 1980;90:661–666.

92. Nager GT. Mastoid and paranasal sinus infections and their relation to the central nervous system. *Clin Neurosurg* 1966;14:288–313.

93. Dawes JDK. The management of frontal sinusitis and its complications. *J Laryngol Otol* 1961;75:297–354.

94. Guibor P. Surgical reconstruction of complications associated with fronto-ethmoid mucocele surgery. *Trans Pa Acad Ophthalmol Otolaryng* 1975;80:454–457.

95. Johnson DL, Markle BM, Wiedermann BL, Hanahan L. Treatment of intracranial abscesses associated with sinusitis in children and adolescents. *J Pediatr* 1988;113:15–23.

96. Oliveira TD, Reimao R, Diament AJ. Intracranial abscesses in

infancy and childhood: report of 40 cases. *Arq Neuropsiquiatr* 1984;42:195–202.

97. Carter BL, Bankoff MS, Fisk JD. Computed tomographic detection of sinusitis responsible for intracranial and extracranial infections. *Radiology* 1983;147:739–742.

98. Zimmerman RA, Bilaniuk LT. CT of orbital infection and its cerebral complications. *AJR* 1980;134:45–50.

99. Weingarten K, Zimmerman RD, Becker RD, Heier LA, Haimes AB, Deck MD. Subdural and epidural empyemas: MR imaging. *AJR* 1989;152:615–621.

100. Luken MG, Whelan MA. Recent diagnostic experience with subdural empyema. *J Neurosurg* 1980;52:764–771.

101. Sadhu VK, Handel SF, Pinto RS, Glass TF. Neuroradiologic diagnosis of subdural empyema and CT limitations. *AJNR* 1980;1:39–44.

102. Dunker RO, Khakoo RA. Failure of computed tomographic scanning to demonstrate subdural empyema. *JAMA* 1981;246:1116–1118.

103. Fairbanks DNF. *Pocket guide to antimicrobial therapy in otolaryngology–head & neck surgery.* Washington, DC: The American Academy of Otolaryngology, 1989;5–11.

104. Brook I. Bacteriologic features of chronic sinusitis in children. *JAMA* 1981;246:967–969.

105. Muntz HR, Lusk RP. Bacteriology of the ethmoid bullae in children with chronic sinusitis. *Arch Otolaryngol* 1991;117:179–181.

106. Brook I, Friedman EM. Intracranial complications of sinusitis in children. A sequela of periapical abscess. *Ann Otol Rhinol Laryngol* 1982;91:41–43.

107. Brook I, Friedman EM, Rodriguez WJ, Controni G. Complications of sinusitis in children. *Pediatrics* 1980;66:568–572.

108. Idriss ZH, Gutman LT, Kronfol NM. Brain abscesses in infants and children: current status of clinical findings, management and prognosis. *Clin Pediatr (Phila)* 1978;17:738–740,745–746.

109. Yang Shu-Yuen. Brain abscess—a review of 400 cases. *J Neurosurg* 1979;55:794–799.

110. Adinoff AD, Cummings NP. Sinusitis and its relationship to asthma. *Pediatr Ann* 1989;18:785–790.

111. Nelson JD. *Pocketbook of pediatric antimicrobial therapy.* Baltimore: Williams & Wilkins, 1990;40–41.

112. Whelan MA, Hilal SK. Computed tomography as a guide in the diagnosis and follow-up of brain abscess. *Radiology* 1980;135:663–671.

113. Rennels MB, Woodward CL, Robinson WL. Medical cure of apparent brain abscesses. *Pediatrics* 1983;72:220–224.

114. Long WD, Meacham WF. Experimental method for producing brain abscess in dogs with evaluation of the effect of dexamethasone and antibiotic therapy on the pathogenesis of intracerebral abscesses. *Surg Forum* 1968;19:437–438.

115. Lyons RE, Enzmann DR, Britt RH. Short-term high-dose corticosteroids in computed tomographic staging of experimental brain abscess. *Neuroradiology* 1982;23:279–284.

116. Newelt EA, Lawrence MS, Blank ND. Effect of gentamicin and dexamethasone on the natural history of the rat *Escherichia coli* brain abscess model with histopathological correlation. *Neurosurgery* 1984;15:475–483.

117. Quartey GR, Johnston JA, Rozdilsky B. Decadron in the treatment of cerebral abscess: an experimental study. *J Neurosurg* 1976;45:301–310.

118. Kourtopoulos H, Holm SE, Norrby SR. The influence of steroids on the penetration of antibiotics into brain tissue and brain abscesses: an experimental study in rats. *Antimicrob Agents Chemother* 1983;11:245–249.

119. Bohl I, Wallenfang R, Bothe H. The effect of glucocorticoids in the combined treatment of experimental brain abscess in cats. In: Schiefer W, Klinger M, Brock M, eds. *Brain abscess and meningitis: subarachnoid hemorrhage-timing problems.* Berlin: Springer-Verlag, 1981;125–133.

120. Schaefer SD, Anderson RG, Carder HM. Epidural mucopyocele: diagnosis and management. *Otolaryngol Head Neck Surg* 1981;89:523–527.

121. Kennedy DW, Josephson JS, Zinreich SJ, Mattox DE, Goldsmith MM. Endoscopic sinus surgery for mucoceles: a viable alternative. *Laryngoscope* 1989;99:885–895.

122. Kahn M, Griebel R. Subdural empyema: a retrospective study of 15 patients. *Can J Surg* 1984;27:283–288.

123. Rosenbaum GS, Cunha BA. Subdural empyema complicating frontal and ethmoid sinusitis. *Heart Lung* 1989;18:199–202.

124. Pott P. *Observations on the nature and consequences of wounds and contusions of the head.* London: Hitch and Howes, 1760;53–58.

125. Thomas JN, Nel JR. Acute spreading osteomyelitis of the skull complicating frontal sinusitis. *J Laryngol Otol* 1977;91:55–62.

126. Feder HM Jr, Cates KL, Cementina AM. Pott puffy tumor: a serious occult infection. *Pediatrics* 1987;79:625–629.

127. Fairbanks DNF, Milmoe GJ. Complications and sequelae: an otolaryngologist's perspective. *Pediatr Infect Dis J* 1985;4:75–78.

128. Wald ER. Special series: management of pediatric infectious diseases in office practice. *Pediatr Infect Dis* 1983;2:61–68.

129. Zinreich SJ. Paranasal sinus imaging. *Otolaryngol Head Neck Surg* 1990;103:863–868.

130. Zinreich SJ, Kennedy DW, Rosenbaum AE, Gayler BW, Kumar AJ. Paranasal sinuses: CT imaging requirements for endoscopic surgery. *Radiology* 1987;163:769–775.

131. Wenig BL, Goldstein MN, Abramson AL. Frontal sinusitis and its intracranial complications. *Int J Pediatr Otorhinolaryngol* 1983;5:285–302.

132. Todd J, Fishaut M, Kapral F. Toxic-shock syndrome associated with phage-group-1 staphylococci. *Lancet* 1978;2:1116–1118.

133. Reingold AL, Shands KN, Dan BB. Toxic-shock syndrome not associated with menstruation: a review of 54 cases. *Lancet* 1982;1:1–4.

134. Wiesenthal AM, Todd JK. Toxic shock syndrome in children aged 10 years or less. *Pediatrics* 1984;74:112–117.

135. Todd JK. Toxic shock syndrome, *Staphylococcus aureus*, and influenza [letter]. *JAMA* 1987;257:3070–3071.

136. Gallo UE, Fontanarosa PB. Toxic streptococcal syndrome. *Ann Emerg Med* 1990;19:1332–1334.

137. Bartter T, Dascal A, Carroll K. "Toxic strep syndrome"—a manifestation of group A streptococcal infection. *Arch Intern Med* 1988;148:1421–1424.

138. Kim YB, Watson DW. A purified group A streptococcal pyrogenic exotoxin: physicochemical and biological properties including the enhancement of susceptibility to endotoxin lethal shock. *J Exp Med* 1970;131:611–628.

139. Bettin KM, Watson DW. Production of pyrogenic exotoxin by groups of streptococci: association with group A. *J Infect Dis* 1979;140:676–681.

140. Johnson LP, L'Italien JJ. Streptococcal pyrogenic type A (scarlet fever toxin) is related to *Staphylococcus aureus* enterotoxin B. *Mol Gen Genet* 1986;203:354–356.

141. Griffith JA, Perkin RM. Toxic shock syndrome and sinusitis—a hidden site of infection. *West J Med* 1988;148:580–581.

142. Jacobson JA, Kasworm EM, Crass BA. Nasal carriage of toxigenic *Staphylococcus aureus* and prevalence of serum antibody to toxic-shock syndrome toxin 1 in Utah. *J Infect Dis* 1986;153:356–359.

143. Osterholm MT, Kelly JA. Toxin and enzyme characterization of *Staphylococcus aureus* isolates from patients with and without toxic-shock syndrome. *Ann Intern Med* 1982;96:937–940.

Subject Index